## A Doctor's Home Cure for Arthritis

obtainable ingredients. Contains full details of a seven-day programme to end arthritis pain and to begin to regain normal use of joints.

Lon

# A Doctor's
# Home Cure
# for Arthritis

## GIRAUD W. CAMPBELL, D.O.
in association with Robert R. Stone

REVISED AND EDITED BY

Jeanette Ewin BA, PhD

Previously revised by
Roger Newman Turner, N.D., D.O., M.R.O.

Thorsons

The website address is: www.thorsonselement.com

and *Thorsons* are trademarks of
HarperCollins*Publishers* Ltd

First published by Parker Publishing Company,
West Nyack, New York

11

© Giraud W. Campbell 2002

Giraud W. Campbell asserts the moral right
to be identified as the author of this work

A catalogue record of this book
is available from the British Library

ISBN-13   978-0-00-713282-9
ISBN-10   0-00-713282-4

Printed and bound in Great Britain by
Clays Ltd, St Ives plc

# Contents

# Introduction to the Third Edition

Dr Giraud W. Campbell's book *A Doctor's Home Cure for Arthritis*, is a classic among self-help guides. Hundreds of thousands of people around the world have found relief from the pain and crippling of arthritis by following his programme of detoxification, diet and gentle exercise. Many more sufferers can benefit from the basic principles Dr Campbell lays down in this easy-to-follow approach to healing swollen and damaged joints. The programme contains no dangerous drugs or the use of strange mechanical devices. It only asks that you choose healthy foods and beverages that contain the nutrients your body needs to repair and restore itself.

This is an exclusion diet. To gain benefits from the Campbell programme, you will trade discomfort and pain for an eating plan that contains no caffeine, alcohol, sugar, or processed foods. Instead, you will enjoy a wealth of delicious fresh food. Getting better depends on you taking action. If red wine and pizza mean more to you than controlling the pain of hot, swollen joints, then that is your choice. If your life is structured around morning coffee and a drink or two before dinner, giving these up may be an impossible sacrifice. Then again, if you sincerely hate the pain, these life-style changes shrink in their importance. It is up to you.

If you are overweight, it is not unusual to experience a healthy loss of a few kilograms while on the Campbell programme. This will help reduce joint pain in the knees and hips. Maintaining a sensible weight takes unnecessary stress off tender joints.

Many people reap rewards from the diet within a few days. People report reduced swelling, less discomfort and better sleep.

More people experience relief from pain within a week of starting the programme. They are surprised to learn that there are more benefits to come. Stay loyal to the diet for a month before you assess its value to you. Most people are amazed by the difference it makes in the way they feel. (One word of caution – people who have been treated with pharmaceuticals containing gold may experience little pain relief from this diet. However, as the basis of a healthy life-style, it will give even them a body more able to withstand infection and the damaging processes of ageing.)

*A Doctor's Home Cure for Arthritis* was first published in 1979. Since then, our understanding of diseases affecting joints has greatly increased, as has our understanding of how foods affect health. By bringing Dr Campbell's programme up-to-date, the publisher decided this edition would help an even greater number of people conquer their arthritis pain. You will find new information about arthritis and diet inserted into the original text in boxes and footnotes, and in the following general section about this debilitating illness.

## About your diet

### Eat a healthy balance of proteins, carbohydrates, and fats

During the past three decades we have learned a great deal about the balance of proteins, fats and carbohydrates needed for a healthy diet. Roughly, the *total number* of *calories* you consume during a day in food and drink should consist of 55–60 per cent from carbohydrate, 15–20 per cent from protein, and 25–30 per cent from fat. (Remember, a gram of fat contains approximately twice the number of calories as a gram of protein or carbohydrate.) Keep the amount of saturated fat in your diet low – about 10 per cent of your total calories – by reducing the amount of red muscle meat in your diet, but do not reduce your total intake much below that mentioned. Enjoy mono-saturated and poly-unsaturated fats instead of saturated fats. Trade extra virgin olive oil, cold-pressed nut oils, duck fat and creamy avocados for beef drippings, hardened margarine and fatty lamb chops. Although low-fat diets (10–15 per cent *total* calories from fat) are fashionable at the moment, they do not provide a healthy balanced diet. Your body needs fat for good health. For example, dietary fat is necessary for the absorption of vitamins A and D needed for healthy bones.

### Include liver in your diet – and consume nutrients the natural way

There is no other source of food as packed full of vital minerals, vitamins and nutritionally important food components as liver. Because the liver is the metabolic dynamo for the body, and performs more metabolic biochemical tasks than elsewhere, vital nutrients are stockpiled here for quick access. That is why it is a central part of the Campbell diet. Other edible organ meats (known as offal) are also rich in nutrients, but none can match liver. In addition to being an excellent source of high quality protein, it contains iron, zinc, vitamin A and B-complex vitamins. It is a top-ranking source of vitamin B12. It is also a good source of co-enzyme Q10, needed for the strong connective tissue found in healthy bone and the effective use of oxygen by the body.

Meats classified as offal include kidneys, sweetbreads (thymus gland and pancreas), heart, tripe (the smooth muscles from the stomach) and brain. Following the discovery of the human form of BSE, the sale of brain, spinal cord and thymus gland have been banned in Britain. (See comments concerning gout on page 190–92.)

## Supplementing your diet

### Fish oil and essential fatty acids help beat arthritis

Our knowledge of essential fatty acids is one of the fasting growing aspects of human nutrition. Over the past several decades we have come to realize that these delicate molecules play a role in almost every function of the human body, including normal tissue growth and the control of inflammation. The two types of essential fatty acids, omega-3 and omega-6, are both needed for good health, and must form a part of any anti-arthritis diet. Omega-6 fatty acids are easily obtained from the nuts and grains in your diet. Oily fish and grasses are good sources of the omega-3 forms of these nutrients. As we eat far fewer of the foods containing omega-3 than omega-6 fatty acids, supplements are needed.

The original Campbell arthritis diet included a daily dietary supplement of cod liver oil, which is rich in vitamins A and D, and also in omega-3 fatty acids. Many medical and nutritional experts believe that pure fish oil is a better choice than cod liver oil, as large doses of vitamin A, taken over a long period of time, can cause toxic side effects. Also, fish oil contains greater amounts of the specific forms of omega-3 fatty acids known to control inflammation. Good sources of pure fish oil were not as plentiful during the late 1970s as they are today. Do not worry about getting adequate amounts of vitamins A and D; they are both found in liver, which is a major food in the Campbell diet. It is safe to take 500mg of fish oil twice a day. Take with food, and if you also take evening primrose supplements, make sure you consume these separate from fish oil as they compete with one another for metabolic pathways in your body.

## Vitamin E and C

Vitamin E is a powerful antioxidant, and is thought to slow the effects of free radicals responsible for the ageing process. Evidence suggests that the oxidative process caused by excessive numbers of free radicals is slowed by the combined action of vitamins E and C. Free radical damage is thought to be a cause of cartilage loss in joints. Studies on patients with osteoarthritis, conducted by the Framingham Osteoarthritis Cohort Study in the United States, have shown a three-fold reduction in the risk of disease progression in people taking moderate amounts of vitamin C (60mg/day). Vitamin E was also shown to slow cartilage degeneration.

Although smaller doses have been shown to be effective, amounts of vitamins C and E that are considered to be safe are:

Vitamin E – 400 international units (i.u.) per day
Vitamin C – 1000 mg per day

## Get all the minerals you need in your diet

Healthy joints and bones depend on the availability of a number of minerals in the diet. These are listed on pages 130–32.

## Control your pain

*Reduce inflammation by avoiding all foods containing gluten*

The Campbell programme works because it is a strict elimination diet, avoiding alcohol, caffeine, refined sugar, and processed foods. It eliminates all foods containing processed grains (mainly wheat), such as bread, pasta, cakes, and thickened sauces. By following this advice, you eliminate from your diet all foods containing gluten (a natural plant protein not used by the human body). Recent research links gluten with coeliac disease, migraine, and increased inflammatory response. As inflammation is the major cause of arthritis pain, eliminating all sources of gluten from the diet is vital: this includes not only wheat, but also oats, barley, and rye. (Although the Campbell diet suggests whole-grain wheat and oat products, these must be avoided.) To avoid eating gluten, build your diet around maize, various types of rice, millet, buckwheat, and some of the more exotic grains, such as quinoa. Remember that by eliminating all processed foods from your diet, such as cakes, canned soups, stock cubes, and bread – all products enhanced by the manufacturers with added gluten – you will eliminate gluten from your diet, and you will feel better for it!

*Be safe when you detox your body*

Eating the right foods is not enough. You must be certain your body's system of elimination is working to rid itself of unwanted chemicals and the waste products from normal metabolism. By following the Campbell diet, you will be drinking plenty of fluid and enjoying enough fresh high-fibre fruit and vegetables to stimulate healthy elimination. In stubborn cases of constipation, Dr Campbell suggests the use of laxatives, and – if these fail – enemas. Enemas should be undertaken with caution. Enemas and colonic irrigation are discouraged by many experts because they feel these practices can upset the delicate tissues of the lower bowel, whose job it is to remove excess fluid from the faeces. By enjoying fresh fruit, and – when necessary – using a gentle laxative, such as lactulose, or one recommended by your chemist, your body will get all the help it needs.

## A word about gout

Gout is a particularly painful form of arthritis that results from the precipitation of uric acid crystals in joints and soft tissues. It occurs when the body is unable to metabolize natural compounts called purines. Heavy drinking and excessive amounts of fatty food were once thought to cause gout, but we now know that alcohol is only a trigger for this condition, and foods as devoid of calories as asparagus can bring on an attack.

Diet plays a big role in controlling gout. If you know you have gout, avoid eating liver and all other offal (organ meats) including thymus and kidney. Also avoid anchovies, sardines, fish roe (caviar), shellfish, asparagus, mushrooms, peas, beans, spinach, rhubarb, and cauliflower.

Good food choices for gout sufferers include eggs, dairy products, and all vegetables with the exception of those listed above. Celery helps clear uric acid from the blood and should be included in your diet two or three times a week, in soups, salads, stews, as 'dips', and in casseroles.

Fish oil, or other food supplements rich in omega-3 essential fatty acids, help control the pain of arthritis by blocking the metabolic processes that cause inflammation.

## Other food sensitivities

Arthritis sufferers find that a surprising number of foods can cause a flare-up of inflammation in arthritic joints. Culprits include *all* citrus fruit, tomatoes, aubergine, box peppers and potatoes. While on the Campbell diet, test yourself to see if you will profit from giving up specific foods not highlighted by his programme. Cut out entirely all those foods mentioned above. After learning to live without toast, coffee, tea, and red wine with pizza, for a few days avoid orange juice, lemon marmalade, tomato salad, moussaka, and mash. If you are sensitive to any of these foods you will experience a noticeable decrease in joint pain and inflammation. To identify exactly which of these foods are culprits in your case, re-introduce them into your diet, one at a time, and see if they cause a flare-up of pain. Wait about 24 hours for results between these tests.

## Cooking tips

*Enjoy organic foods*

Dr Campbell advises you to eat foods that are raw and unprocessed whenever possible. Contamination of food by agricultural chemicals, preservatives, flavour enhancers, artificial colouring, and so on is a bigger problem today than it was in 1979, when *A Doctor's Home Cure for Arthritis* was first published. For that reason, whenever possible search out foods that are organic. When this is not possible, look for sources that contain as few added chemicals as possible. Some farmers specialize in foods guaranteed free from all hormones, antibiotics, pesticides, and preservatives; this form of agriculture is similar to organic, although animals are not housed in the same way. (Even organic farmers use antibiotics when their animals are ill, but these are safe and kept to a minimum.)

*Use your microwave for good flavour and nutrition*

Microwave cooking has received undeserved bad press. Used correctly, these appliances cook fresh food quickly with a reduced loss of many nutrients. Follow the directions provided with your microwave, and enjoy vegetables with texture and colour never achieved with more traditional cooking methods. (Owning a microwave oven tends to encourage the use of processed fast foods. Do not fall into this trap.)

*Use certain canned and frozen foods to make life simpler*

Although Dr Campbell roundly condemns them, there are some canned and frozen foods that can safely be included in your diet. For example, frozen peas and spinach are real convenience foods, and contain more of certain nutrients than are found in fresh produce that was harvested many days before reaching the supermarket shelves. As for canned foods, water-packed beans, corn, chickpeas, or lentils are safe bets; just give them a good rinse before tossing them in a salad, or including them in a casserole.

## Treating arthritis

### Aspirin may cause stomach distress

Many arthritis sufferers are told to take aspirin for relief from arthritis pain and inflammation. However, many people find aspirin causes gastric distress and, when used in large quantities over an extended period of time, may cause damage to the delicate tissues lining the stomach; this may lead to the formation of ulcers. Unfortunately, the same caution pertains to products containing ibuprofen, which can also harm gastric tissue when taken in large amounts. Aspirin and ibuprofen are among drugs classified as non-steroidal anti-inflammatory drugs (NSAID), all of which have the same drawback.

Pain-relief products containing paracetamol are effective alternatives, although people suffering from liver or kidney damage should not use these. It is always best to discuss the products you take for pain management with your doctor.

### Glucosamine sulphate – new hope for arthritis sufferers

Joints occur where two bones meet. To allow movement, the ends of the bones are encased in a fibrous sac that is lubricated with fluid, and the ends of the bones are coated with soft pads of cartilage. In joints affected by this painful illness, the cartilage that cushions the movement of bones against one another is destroyed.

Over the years anti-inflammatory drugs have been manufactured to control the heat, swelling and pain of arthritis, but these pharmaceuticals have been unable to stimulate the re-growth of cartilage. Once damage began there was little that could be done. All that is changing. Remarkable results have been achieved by using a naturally occurring compound called glucosamine sulphate. This is one of the natural constituents of joint tissue. Taken with food in quantities between 500 and 1500mg per day, glucosamine has been demonstrated to have remarkable healing effects on joint cartilage in many cases. (In prolonged use of high doses, mild gastric symptoms may occur.)

### Chondrotin sulphate

Chondrotin sulphate is another compound found in normal joint cartilage that has been shown to help stimulate the rebuilding of healthy joints. It has not been shown to be as effective as glucosamine sulphate, but is thought to work well with it. Many products on the market contain both compounds.

### Methylsulfonylmcthane (MSM)

MSM occurs naturally in body cells, and is thought to play a role in controlling nerve impulses associated with pain. It also appears to help control inflammation. Some experts advise combining MSM and glucosamine sulphate as part of your anti-arthritis regimen of food supplements. However, these supplements should be taken with food, and stopped if there are any signs that gastric pain is associated with their use.

### Dimethyl supfoxide (DMSO)

First used as an industrial solvent, DMSO has found favour as a treatment for a specific form of cystitis, and — more recently — as a treatment for arthritis. Until more research is done on this product, use only with the advice of your doctor or naturopath.

### Nicinamide (a form of vitamin $B_3$)

Scientific research has shown that, when taken in high dosages, this vitamin helps control pain. Do not use this treatment without being monitored by your doctor, as high dosages may have side-effects.

### S-adenosylmethionine (SAMe)

SAMe is a form of the amino acid methionine, and has been shown to have an effect on pain similar to that of ibuprofen. This should not be taken by people with manic-depressive illness.

### Herbs

Boswellia and cayenne extracts are plant products that have been shown to help arthritis sufferers when used according to directions.

Boswellia is a treatment used in traditional medicine as practised in India, and is thought to block the biological processes leading to inflammation. When cayenne extract as applied to the skin as a cream, it appears to block pain messages before they reach the brain.

# A Word from Dr Campbell

In this book I provide you with the treatment for arthritis that has cured hundreds of sufferers.

It has not mattered whether these patients of mine were old or young.

It has not mattered in what part of the body they had the arthritis.

It has not mattered whether the doctor who referred them to me said it was caused by an infection, or what type of arthritis he said they had.

It has not mattered whether they were still getting around or whether they were bedridden.

It has not mattered whether they had arthritis for six months, six years, or longer.

Their arthritis was cured or significantly improved.

Yours can be, too.

What does matter is that you want to get rid of your arthritis badly enough that you are willing to follow the exact but simple procedures in this book. These have to do largely with diet and elimination.

When my patients have followed these procedures, here is what they found:

- Heat and swelling in the affected joints was eased within one week.
- Pain was relieved, in most cases eliminated, in two weeks or less.

11

- More normal movement of the affected parts in the vast majority of cases was enjoyed in three weeks or less.
- X-rays revealed progress in the restoration of damaged bone structure in three to six months.

Now these are not special cases. They are average arthritic sufferers. A mother, bedridden for months because of her arthritis, does housework again. An engineer, on crutches for a year, tosses them aside after three weeks. A grandmother, previously crippled by arthritis, discards her wheelchair ... to cite just a few cases. There are many more set out in this book.

Once cured, if you do not want to be confronted by the spectre of a pain-racked arthritic life again, you will have to remain vigilant. Ease up on the regimen and you are likely to be once again a candidate for an arthritis nightmare.

Unfortunately, there are some cases that this regimen of diet, improved circulation, and elimination cannot help. Arthritis sufferers who have had extensive gold treatments do not usually respond to this natural therapy. Neither do those patients respond who have had extensive drug or chemical treatment. Apparently, changes in the blood or metabolism occur which impede this cure.

This arthritis cure is so simple it has been largely ignored up until now.

It needs a voice.

I thank the publisher of this book for making it possible for you to hear this voice. And I appeal to all of you who may be cured of arthritis through this book to share that experience with your doctor so that other sufferers may also benefit.

*Giraud W. Campbell D.O.*

# CHAPTER 1

# Proof That Arthritis *Can* Be Cured

"I had terrible pains in my left shoulder and upper arm ... All I could do was hold my arm and walk. If I sat down a while, the ache became unbearable ..."

Millions of arthritis sufferers know exactly what this person is talking about. But how many would understand what this person means when she says:

"Within three weeks I was without pain and could go to work feeling my old self again ... jump out of bed and feel alive."

A sudden 'remission'? An unexplainable cure? Well, then, how about this woman's case history:

"I found myself almost a cripple, unable to walk without pain. I tried several doctors. Aspirin, gold injections, cortisone drugs – nothing seemed to help. I kept getting continually worse, endured constant pain, and had to be pulled up from a chair; helped at every step ..."

Then, after four years of suffering, this person went on a new arthritis treatment presented to you in the pages ahead. The following change took place:

"I am now able to stand up straight, move about without pain, get a good night's sleep and do housework. I enjoy life again!"

How would you feel if you were a doctor prescribing a cure for a disease and having success after success – while Doctors of Medicine (M.D.s) were declaring adamantly that *arthritis is incurable*?

It's pretty frustrating, especially when you think about those millions who are now crippled and suffering from arthritis and who could instead enjoy life again because ...

*Arthritis can be cured.*

*Arthritis is being cured.*

People who have become resigned to life in a wheelchair are walking and enjoying pain-free, drug-free days once again.

## Improvement of bone structure

As I was explaining this treatment to a medical colleague of mine he said: "Wait a minute, wait a minute! You don't mean arthritis can be cured. You mean that the pain and the inflammation of the joints can be relieved. But the bones...?"

Yes, *the bone structure in arthritis can be improved too*. I showed this doctor X-rays to prove it. He examined them with genuine amazement. He was looking at proof that kneecaps were un-fusing themselves, compressed vertebrae were regenerating, bony overgrowth was being reduced and its proliferation checked and absorbed.

Then he was ready to listen to the cure for arthritis.

## The key to arthritis cure

After I outlined the basic steps, he threw his hands up. "You mean to say you get people to stay on a rigid regimen (diet) like that?"

"I don't. But the pains of arthritis keep the sufferer on the diet beam."

(He changed the subject to rising prices and taxes.)

The healing arts form a strange family – chiropractic, naturopathy, osteopathy, conventional medicine. You would think practitioners in these various healing arts would exchange views, findings and successes in the interests of humanity. Instead, I find there is non-cooperation between them, and quite some competition.*

Arthritis is being cured now largely through diet. Diet is not popular among medical doctors (the M.D.s). Even obesity is treated by them most frequently with multi-coloured pills, albeit some aimed at curbing appetite.

* There are strong indications of these attitudes changing to a spirit of cooperation between all medical disciplines. *Editor*

The blessings of an end of arthritis are yours when you follow the programmes on the pages ahead. It is so natural, so easy, so largely self-administered and so easily diet-oriented. It will very likely be skipped over by the medical profession for some time to come as they continue their search for a virus, bacterium, or other type of microorganism or else an unbalance that causes the body to attack itself – and of course, for the medicine to counteract it. Rheumatoid arthritis is called an auto-immune disorder because of the tendency for the immune system to damage the body's own tissues.

Every medical researcher wants to be a Lister or a Pasteur or Banting to gain the kudos which comes from making an astounding discovery that leads to a magic bullet cure. But there is no glory for the founder of a treatment that involves eating certain foods and giving up others. Arthritis is so easily prevented and so easily cured that it warrants no Nobel prizes.

One of the problems that both the Arthritis Foundation in the US and the Arthritis and Rheumatism Council in the UK have wrestled with in their attempts to raise research money is that arthritis is neither contagious nor fatal. It therefore lacks the public motivating power of cancer, for example, to launch an all-out publicized attack.

In effect, the medical community says to let the millions suffer from arthritis another day – there are lives to be saved from other more threatening diseases.

And suffer they do from arthritis.

## Beware of quack remedies

Another problem that has, in effect, closed the public's receptivity to a cure for arthritis is that cruel hoaxes are being played on arthritic sufferers by those who seek to exploit pain for personal gain. These quacks siphon hundreds of millions of pounds a year from the already strained coffers of arthritic sufferers with their 'treatments,' 'cures,' and 'devices.'

Meanwhile, the cure lies in your own kitchen and on your own dining-room table at no expense and perhaps at even a cost saving.

## Expect a 'miracle'!

While the search for a cure for arthritis goes on, hundreds, for a fact, are being cured of this crippling painful disease.

While scientists theorize about the high white blood-cell count or the low red blood-cell count, hundreds of arthritic sufferers are emerging from their ordeal with a normal blood count.

While scientists are debating over bacteria, viruses and mycoplasma, the disease is abating for those who eliminate the wrong foods.

While statisticians were recording 250,000 new sufferers each year, hundreds were being taken off the crippled list on Long Island, NY, where the author had his practice.

While books, films, and TV documentaries relate sadly moving stories of people losing their fight with arthritis, others are winning that fight.

While new salicylates, like aspirin, are perfected to relieve those whose lives are destined to be plagued by arthritic pain, that pain is gone forever within seven days for those who eat in a special way and follow the guidance in this book.

While medical 'authorities' affirm adamantly that there is no specific diet effective in arthritis, thus keeping millions in its bondage, hundreds are gaining permanent freedom *via diet*.

While patients are being injected with placentas (the material of after-birth), with ACTH (a hormone compound) and with gold and other chemical compounds, only to find that temporary relief is the most they can expect, others are treating themselves with delicious, nutritional food and enjoying permanent cure.

I confess right here and now that I cannot help those who have had extensive gold treatments and who have undergone blood changes because of extended drug or chemical treatment.

The rest of you:

- Expect a 'miracle.'
- Expect your pain to start diminishing from the start with the programmes in this book.
- Expect no need for aspirin or other pain relievers in a week or ten days.
- Expect a continuing improvement in your joint mobility.
- Expect a gradual restoration of damaged bone.
- Expect your return to a normal life without arthritic pain.

## The price of an arthritis cure

At what price, you ask?

The price of cure from the crippling effects of arthritis is:

- A willingness to give up certain foods that you may have been eating almost daily all your life.
- A willingness to adopt as a steady diet certain foods that you rarely eat now.
- A willingness to undergo a few minutes of effort in the interest of internal hygiene.
- A willingness, in cases of long-term damage, to undergo some mild physical therapy.
- A willingness to devote a few minutes a day to gentle physical routines aimed at accelerating neuro-muscular and joint restoration.

Now, this may be too much of a price to pay for an arthritis cure. There is just a little more you should consider:

- Are you willing to give up coffee and tea?
- Are you willing to accept the fact that bread and all other flour products are bad news for arthritis sufferers?
- Are you willing to give up soft drinks and hard drinks – at least until you are cured and then to imbibe them only at the risk of a return of your arthritis pains?
- Are you willing to give up canned and other processed foods, especially ice cream and other sweet concoctions?

To those who hesitate conforming to the above points, I promise assistance in the habit-breaking department. Breaking long-held habits by sheer willpower, even with the tremendous reward of an end to arthritis, can still be a super-human task. It can be made easier through a simple process known as re-conditioning yourself.

To those who balk altogether, to those who will not follow simple habit-changing instructions, I say, "Read no further." Apparently for you the price of cure is too high. No hard feelings, but we have come to the parting of the ways.

The rest of you who are glad to be healed of your arthritis follow me for the rest of this book.

## Some case histories

### The case of Mrs A. S.

Mrs A. S. was 65. She had been married 45 years, had raised four children, was a grandmother 16 times, a great-grandmother four times.

Suddenly the enjoyment of the youngsters was interrupted. She began to experience pains and stiffness in her arms and legs.

Let her tell you the story of what followed:

"My family physician diagnosed my illness as arthritis and treated me for a period of one month. Seeing no progress, he referred me to an arthritis specialist. After thoroughly examining my heart, shoulder and lung X-rays, the specialist stated I did not have arthritis, but my problem was frozen shoulders. He then referred me to an orthopaedic specialist who, after re-examining the X-rays, referred me to a therapist who gave me six treatments. Noting I was not being relieved by these treatments, he directed me to a medical centre for cobalt treatments. After I had received six of these cobalt treatments with no relief, he sent me back to the orthopaedic doctor, who said he was sorry, but he could not help me.

A friend, who worked as a hospital laboratory technician, suggested I go to an arthritis clinic. The clinic diagnosed my case as rheumatoid arthritis and said there was no cure and no help.

Discouraged and bewildered, I went home and finally became bedridden with severe pain throughout my body: my shoulders, arms, knees, wrists, fingers and feet. I was thus bedridden for 15 weeks."

This story really has a happy ending. I visited Mrs A. S. at her home. So let's hear the rest of her story ...

"Imagine my happy and encouraged surprise when Dr Campbell told me, if I would faithfully follow diet instructions, he would have me walking sufficiently to be able to come to his office (with some help). This was on a Wednesday, and by the following Saturday I was able to go to his office."

Read what happened a year later:

"I am able to arise in the morning, make my own bed, walk up and down stairs, go out to dine, visit friends and go shopping in the company of my husband."

To me as a doctor it's a familiar ending. I see it every day. To others it's a miracle. This woman suffered for less than a year. The average arthritic person suffers for more than ten years, turning what could be golden years into agonized ones.

The pain of arthritis is torment. It gnaws, grates, and rankles. Joints become heated and inflamed. Movement is often excruciating. The distress can be acute, sharp, piercing. Or it can be achy, throbbing, and consuming.

It is a cruel pain in that it subsides just as you feel you can get used to it. You feel blessed relief. Then it comes back stronger than ever.

It is a desolating pain because it defies courage and lays it low. The more the resolve to move despite the pain, the more harrowing the effort. It leaves you no choice but to avoid the throes of movement and remain immobile and alone.

**Walter M's Case**

"I was in agony." This is a 52-year-old man, Walter M., recalling his ordeal. "Something was wrong with my spine in the region of my shoulder blades. I had visited medical men – one a general practitioner, the other a neuro-surgeon – and I could not obtain relief. The neuro-surgeon prescribed traction treatments which did not ease my pain. The condition was so bad that I could not sleep in bed. The pain was such that I had to sleep in an upright position at the dining-room table. I slept by sitting on a pillow and drooping myself across the table on another pillow."

This was pain indeed. Can you imagine what happens to a person deep inside when pain such as this is prolonged?

Fortunately for this man, our paths crossed. In two weeks his arthritis of the spine had improved under my guidance to the point where he could once again sleep in comfort.

## A case which inspired a cure

When I was a young intern, just graduated from college, some 40 short years ago, I was assigned to a very nice lady suffering from general acute rheumatoid arthritis. She was only 48 years old, yet one of the most pathetic cases I was to see for many years.

This patient was a wheelchair case. Her knees would not bend. Every joint in her body was racked with constant pain, swelling and heat. To put a bed pan under her, which was done as infrequently as possible, caused excruciating pain. This woman had great confidence in me and she felt sure I could cure her. Her pleading eyes made me very uncomfortable because at that time I knew of nothing that could help her.

I was grateful when, after two months on this assignment, I was transferred to the hospital emergency ward. This meant that I wouldn't be embarrassed each time I saw her in her room and she, in turn, couldn't have lost confidence in me since she would assume that I didn't have enough time to spend with her to cure her.

Today I welcome these cases. Their relief is rapid and dramatic. The pain my patients lose is due in large part to the pain this lady did not lose. It is the indelible impression she left on my mind – her utter helplessness and her great confidence in me – which drove me throughout the years to perfect a successful treatment. I can still see her. How I wish I had known then what I know today.

## The real cause of arthritis

There are over 25 million pet dogs in the United States and almost as many cats. Despite the reassuring advertising, the foods these pets eat are not adequately nutritious. As a result, veterinarians enjoy thriving practices treating dogs and cats that get certain nationally advertised pet food but nevertheless suffer from bone and joint diseases as well as skin, eye, and coat troubles.

Are the pets being exploited?

Are the food manufacturers taking advantage of our dumb animals?

The answer is "no."

The pets are actually getting a better deal than we humans are!

The reason is that the natural instincts of dogs and cats prevent them from eating the kind of synthetic and adulterated products that we blindly consume, the foods that look so good, take no time to prepare, and keep forever.

Pet-food manufacturers can't get away with half the things that human-food manufacturers do.

Man is not so smart after all.

He smokes despite the pollution it brings to his lungs and the threat of pulmonary disease.

He consumes soft drinks, colas, tea, coffee, and alcoholic beverages, – trading a few minutes of physical pleasure for years of depleted health.

He eats dead food – devitalized, demineralized, devitaminized foods that have been bleached, leached, and refined of all nature's goodness, and he substitutes instead a few synthetic 'enriching' ingredients and a hundred other chemical additives that gradually pollute his entire system.

Too bad it does not catch up with him immediately in an acute case of stomachache.

Anything that causes that immediate reaction is banned. If it creeps up on us over weeks, months, and years, then it's acceptable.

The poisons we eat in processed foods are said to be "within tolerable limits."

Is arthritis a tolerable limit?

Arthritis is largely the product of our unwholesome eating habits.

Correct these habits and the cure begins!

Correct these habits? That's a laugh. Who can break even a simple habit? It's impossible for most people. Little unwanted mannerisms go on and on. Smoking goes on and on. Most of us live by daily routine. Habits are comfortable. Change is difficult.

Habits break easily only when the load of pain and problem they produce becomes heavy enough.

Arthritis is heavy enough.

### A War Veteran's Case

A veteran of World War II suffered much longer. Here is how he describes his ordeal:

"I would like to record my experience with arthritis for the benefit of other victims of this terrible disease.

"I was discharged from the army in 1945. Shortly thereafter, I began to experience pains in my lower back and shooting pains down the back of my legs. It got really bad and so I sought the services of some local doctors. No relief was obtained. As time went by, I felt the Veteran's Hospital should be the place to go, especially since the disease entered my entire spine and became even more painful. Motion became extremely difficult and pain was constant. I spent four years as an out-patient of the Veteran's Hospital, visiting them twice a week, with no relief. It was now diagnosed as Marie Strümpell's Disease.

"Later, I came under the service of an arthritic specialist, who treated me over a period of *nine years* with all kinds of medications and injections. The disease steadily grew worse. I became more crippled. My spine, at this time, had practically fused solid. Pain was more intense and by now it was continuous, day and night, with no relief.

"At this point, I heard of Dr Giraud Campbell and went to see him. He immediately put me on a diet. This was the first time anyone had mentioned anything about foods; what to eat and what not to eat. I was in such pain, I was willing to try anything.

"To my amazement, within two weeks, the pain decreased at least 50 per cent. Stiffness persisted for a long period of time, yet I was able to walk better. No longer did I have to walk like a turtle, with my head stretched out, in order to be able to see where I was going. Nevertheless, my spine was bent forward in a semi-circle, which was gradually straightened so that I no longer walk in the characteristic posture of a Marie Strümpell's Disease victim. The diet together with prescribed exercises and Dr Campbell's treatments brought about this improvement.

"This is a remarkable achievement. I only wish I had come under Dr Campbell's care some time when the disease first started. I would never have had to experience the excruciating pain I did over the years, nor would I have had to become deformed.

"Other victims of this dreaded disease should know that relief and cure is readily available. They should never have to go through the horrors I went through. This simple treatment system should be available to all."

## Where arthritis begins

There was a time when we ate farm fresh food. Farm-to-market roads brought fresh produce to the table in matter of days. Soil was rich. Fresh food brimmed with vitamins, minerals, and other nutrients.

As the soil became depleted, chemicals were added. They helped. But not as much as the composted waste that some farmers were returning to their soil. The character of food changed.

Enter the food processors' impact on our eating habits.

Did you ever read the label on a can or box of processed foods? The big chemical names are too hard to read and pronounce. Too bad the chemicals are not just as hard to swallow There are also harmful ingredients hiding behind such innocent-sounding words as 'flavouring,' 'modified,' 'enriched,' and 'colouring.' These are just as insidious and dangerous.

Behind these words stands a growing, flourishing industry that uses the power of advertising, public relations, and lobbying to promote the concept that natural foods contain impurities and poisons, while their manufactured products are pure and healthful. They have succeeded for decades, but ...

Slowly but surely the public is beginning to react. Thanks to people like Rachel Carson, Robert Rodale, Carlson Wade, Dr M. O. Garten, Dr A. Chase, and other brave nutritionists and naturopaths we are beginning to see through the food processors' subterfuges and to understand what is happening.

Did you know that a famous firm in the photography business is in the food-processing business? They sell 'monoesters.' These monoesters are said by the manufacturer to make "dehydrated potatoes even better than the homemade kind." Monoesters, they say, "assure a smooth, mouthwatering consistency." Undoubtedly they do. But do we know anything more about their effects – especially long-term effects?

Did you know that a famous manufacturer of explosives is in the food-processing business? They give us many types of cellulose gum to lengthen the shelf-life of bakery products and to thicken gravies, soups and sauces. They advertise that these cellulose gums make the food taste better. I wonder how it affects the ability of the body to derive vitality from the food.

Acceptance in the market place seems to be the motivating factor. If the effects of additives are not acutely detrimental, who is going to take the time and spend the money to determine their long-term effects?

Imitation chicken flavour, imitation beef flavour, imitation peanut flavour – all 'better than the real thing.' We live in a food world of genuine imitations.

Only our body remains unfooled by these claims of benefits.

Who is to blame? The stockholders of these companies, the board of directors, the foremen, the workers? No. We, the consumers, are to blame! We ask for it. We seek the easier, the quicker, and we sound our own death knell all the quicker.

Are we trapped in the supermarket of super-processed, superrefined foods? Or are there alternatives?

Fortunately, there is still a way out.

If there were no way out, I would be offering a theoretical cure for arthritis that no one could take advantage of.

The way out, on the pages ahead, ends the massive doses of pollution of various kinds that we are administering to our body. Also, through a natural cleansing process, it helps undo the pollution effects of past years.

You, the arthritic sufferer must understand right here and now that your *tolerance* for nutritional pollution has evidenced itself to be less than non-sufferers. You are over the critical point because you suffer from arthritis.

You must reverse the process if you want to get rid of your arthritis, by ridding yourself of the effects of self-pollution.

## Signs that point the way for you

Every day our newspapers and magazines point to a change. Recently I scanned a community newspaper. At the top of one page was the headline "Inventor Develops Better Way to Bake Bread."The item told of a new patent to prolong shelf life of baked goods using "a novel class of chemical compounds" termed 'micro-crystalline stearyl fumaric compounds.'The patent is assigned to a famous pharmaceutical company.

Directly below this five-column story was a one-column item titled "Club Goes Organic," about a local garden club devoting its next meeting to a study of organic gardening and earth management.

I shudder at the economic power of the giant pharmaceutical firm. How little power had the small club by comparison! And also, how much interest do you think the garden-club story generated?

## Getting back to nature

Dr Weston Price, in his book, *Nutrition and Physical Degeneration*, tells the story of two American prospectors who were flown into a remote part of Canada to survey an area for its mineral content. The plane had to deposit them 100 miles from their destination.

They planned to hike the remaining distance on foot over difficult terrain.

In a short time, one of the men developed burning in his eyes followed by blurred vision. Finally, he couldn't see any more, so his companion left him at a marked spot with ample food for two months and went to seek help. The victim became worse. Three days later, when an Indian came upon the now blind man, the Indian recognized the trouble as a food deficiency. He caught some brook trout, then he stood by and insisted that the prospector eat them raw, including the eyes. By the time the rescuers came back, the man's sight had been restored and he was able to return to 'civilization' under his own power.

We call American Indians 'primitive,' yet they knew what foods to eat to stay healthy. They did not die of heart disease, diabetes, cancer, or hardening of the arteries as we moderns do.

When the French explorer Jacques Cartier made his famous voyage to Montreal, Canada, a great many of his crew developed a dreaded disease, fatal in those days, which today we know as scurvy – due to vitamin C deficiency. These crew members, some 30 odd, were put to shore to survive as best they could.

The chief of the Tuscarora tribe, a member of the Iroquois nation at that time, noting the plight of the crew members, ordered his warriors to feed them young spruce shoots, which today we know are loaded with vitamin C. When Cartier returned some years later, he was amazed to see his motley crew in fine health and the fathers of many healthy children.

Nature seems to be abounding with miraculous cures. But this is an illusion! It just seems that way. Actually we create a civilization abounding with unnatural causes of problems. When we return to nature, these problems disappear.

The cure for arthritis is in a way a return to nature. It is a return to basic natural foods that provide the body with its nutritional needs without the unnatural additives and the 'civilized' depletion that twentieth-century living seems to mandate.

We are a product of our environment. But we wanted to change nature, and so we have changed ourselves – but not to our health advantage.

Some of these changes are great. They give us comforts and widen our horizons with a multiplicity of experiences.

Some of us change slower than others. It is more difficult for some of us to adjust to new stresses, to new tensions, to new anxieties – but none can adjust to new food additives.

## The price of food technology

During World War I, some 25 per cent of the young men called to the colours had to be rejected because they were physically or mentally unfit. About 25 years in food technology later, some 50 per cent of our prime young men had to be rejected – even with lower physical requirements. Had these requirements remained unchanged, the rejections would have topped 70 per cent!

Arthritis is only one malfunction of the body now manifesting in even our younger men. The full list reads like a medical dictionary.

Why has this been happening? Is our longer life expectancy to be marred by illness and disease? Are we moving forwards or backwards?

### Health secret of the Hunzas

In West Pakistan there is a region which was formerly an independent kingdom. It is known as Hunza. The Hunzas live to over 100 years of age. Sickness like cancer, heart attacks, arthritis, the childhood diseases, are rare. Even mental health is on a high level with no juvenile delinquency, no crime, and hardly ever a divorce.

Those who have visited, studied, and reported back on the Hunzas will differ on the probable reasons behind their extraordinarily high level of health. Some say it is due to their genuine love of their fellow man. Others say that it is due to their inner peace. Others that it is due to their natural diet. Of course, all three are vital factors, but there is more to know about the Hunzas.

Consider the Hunzas diet. It is largely fresh vegetables, both the leafy and root kind; whole grains; fruit and berries, both fresh and sun-dried; butter, cheese, and other dairy products.

Hunzas care not if their milk turns sour. They drink it that way and they drink their buttermilk that way. They consider it a natural and complete food.

In recent years, as better communication has brought the benefits of civilization to the Hunzas, their health has started to decline appreciably. The younger generation of Hunzas are increasingly prone to the same degenerative diseases as their Western counterparts – giving further emphasis to Dr Campbell's argument.

### What has happened to our commercial milk?

What happens with our milk by contrast?

First, our cows graze on depleted pastures and are themselves at a lesser state of natural health than their Hunza counterparts. We take our cows' milk and we homogenize it.

We are taught that homogenizing is good. It permits milk to stand around longer without turning sour. It prevents milk and cream from separating so we don't have to go to the trouble of shaking the bottle each time.

But here is the price we pay for less-frequent deliveries to the grocer and less muscle work by ourselves:

The process of homogenization consists of putting milk under high pressure and elevated temperature. This changes the raw protein in milk and makes it less nutritional. It destroys an enzyme known as phosphatase which is necessary for the utilization of calcium and phosphorus. It destroys some of the vitamin B and most of the vitamin C.

Up to the early 1900s milk was a complete food. It was whole milk. It was not skimmed, boiled, powdered, condensed, pasteurized, or homogenized. Occasionally it was certified – a means of insuring through controlled-feeding conditions and testing that the milk was highly nutritious, hygienic, and fresh. But it was not processed.

Your best health buy is certified organic milk; if that is not available, choose non-homogenized pasteurized milk. Pasteurized milk is safe because it has been gently heated to kill potentially dangerous bacteria. This has little effect on its nutritional content. Unless you can obtain certified milk directly from a farm you know you can trust, drink pasteurized milk.

Milk is homogenized to prevent the cream separating from the watery, protein-rich portion. Both homogenized and non-homogenized milk are safe to drink.

Semi-skimmed is the most highly processed of all forms of milk. Removing the cream from milk produces skimmed milk. This is a simple matter and adds little in the way of processing. By contrast, semi-skimmed milk is first skimmed and then enriched with cream. Strict standards determine exactly how much cream is reintroduced into a batch of skimmed milk.

Multiply the changes that have occurred in milk a few hundred times and you begin to have a picture of what we have done to the balance of nature within our own bodies. It is little wonder that more of us don't have arthritis and the host of degenerative diseases and metabolic imbalances that keep our doctors busy and our hospitals full.

There is little raw milk available to urban and even suburban areas. But there are ways to reduce the deprivation to which we are subjecting our body and to compensate for past abuse.

The way is not easy, but the results are immediate and magnificent as the following will show you.

## To sum up the cure for arthritis

As you have read in previous pages, the price for getting rid of your arthritis might be quite high for you to pay, but the price is not in money. I have been trying to give this warning to you slowly and gently and I am confident you are beginning to get the message.

- *No*, you are not going to have to buy a score of gadgets and go through any physical hocus-pocus.
- *No*, you are not going to have to force yourself into swirling pools or diathermy or similar physical coddling.

- *No,* you are not going to have to take bigger and better pills, temporarily numbing your arthritic pains.

*Simpler and worse than that!*

You are going to have to give up some of the things that you have been eating and drinking and liking all your life.

For some of you this is a bitter pill indeed.

To you I say it need not be a permanent sacrifice. As soon as you are free of arthritis you may restore some of these products if you still feel the need for them.

If you want to enjoy permanent cure, however and if you want to have arthritic bone damage disappear in the years ahead, you had better anticipate a new way of life. Take Mrs M. W. Did she go back to her old ways once she was free of heat, swelling, and pain? Mrs M. W. found adjusting to a new way of eating far less painful than arthritis. She adopted this new way of eating permanently. She enjoyed steady improvement. The reward was a normal life.

She gave up some pleasant tastes and some familiar feelings in her mouth. They were difficult for her to give up, but in return she was out of her prison of arthritis pain within a few short days, and enjoyed a steady restoration of glorious normal living.

Is your body ready for these types of amazing rewards? And is your mouth ready to pay the price for ridding yourself of the agonies and tortures caused by the ravages of arthritis? Only you, the arthritis sufferer, can make this vital decision.

## For your action

Re-affirm your willingness to pay the 'price' spelled out on page 17. Go down each of the five points and weigh them against the burden of arthritis. Condition yourself to accept extreme changes in your eating habits – and to expect a 'miracle' of freedom from arthritis.

# CHAPTER 2

# How to Reverse the Cause of Arthritis and Begin the Cure

You will see in this chapter just what arthritis is and why you have to

- purify your body of accumulated poisons, and
- cut off further intake of poison in order to begin the cure.

## Action for your health in your own kitchen

Most of us seldom give a thought to the nutritional value of the foods we buy or to the dangers of chemical additives they contain.

Nutrition seems to be a vague science. It is full of contradictions. What helps some people hurts others. One man's meat is another man's poison. One man's cup of tea is another man's cup of hemlock.

Your poisons are prepared foods and processed foods.

Your poisons are packed desserts.

Your poisons are canned soups, canned fruits, canned meats, canned vegetables, canned fish, canned poultry.

Your poisons are cake, candy, and ice cream.

Your poisons are certain meats.

Your poisons are packaged cereals.

Your poisons are bakery products, spaghetti and pastas, refined rice, noodles, pizza.

Your poisons are coffee, tea, and soft drinks.

Your poisons are jams, jellies, sugar, and artificial sweeteners.

Your poisons are imitation dairy products and other foods fabricated, imitated, altered, or semi-prepared by man.

Your poisons are wine, beer and liquor.

"What's there left to eat?" you say.

There are fresh fruits, garden fresh vegetables, delicious fish, and selected meats. There are natural cheeses, eggs, nuts, and natural sweeteners.

Which of these two would you choose? –

Apple pie à la mode topped with severe arthritic pain, heat, and swelling; or, fresh, raw, mixed vegetable salad including avocado, parsley, watercress, and endive enjoyed with a dash of zestful, absolutely pain-free living.

Need I say more?

Go to your kitchen today. If you live alone, toss out all prepared and manufactured foods. Kiss them goodbye.

Make room for an arthritis-free tomorrow.

If you live with your family or a room-mate, divide up the kitchen so that certain areas are yours. You have *your* own vegetable bin, *your* fruit bowl, *your* section in the refrigerator.

You won't need much shelf space. Shelves are where one stores food that is processed to last almost indefinitely. The cans, the boxes, and the jars.

The processing consists of taking out the germ and essence of the food, the living seed of it, so that even the simplest forms of life – mould, insects, etc. – cannot find anything sustaining in it. *Much less can human beings*!

If you put a certain food on a shelf and nothing happens to it, you should suspect it of not being very nutritive. Of course, there are exceptions like dry seeds and nuts – also, some whole foods like whole, fresh, ground oats that must be vacuum-packed. But, by and large, shelf life has been the 'big deal' for food preservatives and food processing.

On the other hand, you will need to hog your refrigerator space. 'Alive' foods keep better when cool. You will want plenty of space for heads of lettuce, asparagus, cauliflower, most varieties of squash, corn, all kinds of beans, green peppers, leeks, scallions, spinach.

Some vegetables like beets, egg plant, carrots, and onions will keep fresh in a cupboard vegetable bin. So will brown rice and wild rice (white rice is taboo).

You will need refrigeration space, too, for fresh poultry like chicken, duck, squab, goose, and turkey that are raised in a natural environment.

Make room for delicious cuts of lamb, pork, and veal.

Make lots of room for fresh fish, any type that is brought fresh to your area: striped bass, cod, flounder, red snapper, sea bass, fluke, lobster, shrimp, crabs both soft and hard shelled, oysters, mussels, fresh salmon, fresh tuna, halibut, and many more.

Make room for those kinds of fresh fruit that need refrigeration, like blueberries, raspberries, strawberries, plums, nectarines.

Of course, you'll need big fruit bowls for the bananas, apples, pears, cherries, etc. You'll need bowls for the nuts and jars for the seeds.

You are not going to starve after all, are you?

## Fast work in knocking out arthritis

Remember what the little boy replied when his horrified mother asked him why he was banging his head against the wall: "It feels so good when I stop."

You've been banging your body against a stone wall, figuratively speaking, for a long time. It's going to feel magnificent to stop.

When you do, your body will begin to cure itself.

That natural curative power has been there right along, but you have been getting ahead of it. It's not your fault really. But the food that has been easiest to buy, quickest to prepare, and sweetest to the taste buds has been put into your body faster than your body can rid itself of the unnatural, unwanted, detrimental-in-the-long-run ingredients.

There has been a compounding effect: While you have been putting arthritis-causing (among other diseases) impurities into your body, you have also been depriving your body of the health-giving nutrients that provide the body with what it needs to heal, recharge, and renew itself for good health.

The body is first attacked, and then asked to defend itself with one arm tied behind its back.

In a way, arthritis sufferers are fortunate that the poison barrage is coming by way of the food they eat. How easy that is to correct compared to the growing rates of illness due to impure air, impure water, radiation, and other environmental factors that will sooner or later make this planet uninhabitable if not corrected or controlled!

With food, you can still exercise selectivity in the market. But there's nothing you will be able to do in the coming so-called atomic age to protect the cells of your body from the disruptive action of ionizing radiation that emanates silently, odour-free, invisible, and continuously from nuclear sources.

You are the master of your own destiny foodwise as long as there is fresh unprocessed meat, poultry, fish, and produce available to you.

*You can end your arthritis if you want to!*

Air is getting more attention than food or water in our newly health-orientated society. Air pollution may well deserve this priority. Lung cancer may soon be caused as much by breathing as by smoking. What options will we have then?

- Be glad there is something you can do about the pain and misery of arthritis besides prolong your ability to live with it through aspirin and other palliatives or 'nerve blocks'.
- Be glad that you have a choice.
- Be glad there are steps you can take to end the pain and misery of arthritis.
- Be glad those steps are as close as your own kitchen!

## How to begin the purification process

Since arthritis is analogous to a pollution of the body, we must not only stop that polluting but we must do what we can to eliminate the poisons.

34

If a power plant receives more demand, it supplies more. But if it becomes overloaded, it supplies nothing. Most arthritics are constipated. Their organs of elimination have become overloaded.

It is said that Methuselah lived 960 years, Noah 950 years, Adam 930 years. Can you imagine them living that long if they were constipated!

The second part of the arthritis cure is the restoration of your body's organs of elimination. These include not only the bowels but also the kidneys, the skin, and the lungs.

When one of these organs becomes blocked or overloaded, there is an increase of load on the other organs. Often they cannot handle it properly and the body in its infinite wisdom finds its own internal garbage cans.

Did you know where they are? They are easy to find. Just follow the aches and pains.

### Your organs of elimination

If your bowels are so blocked that it is taking longer than it should to eliminate poisons, then you had better do something about it right now. Following are the reasons why:

If *bowels* do not function as they should, the liquid waste from the delayed faecal material must be reabsorbed into your body. It is packed up by the blood stream, carried through the circulation system, and brought to kidneys, skin, and lungs.

In a minute, I am going to give you a simple test to determine just how long poisons are remaining in your large bowel. But first let's see the chain reaction that takes place when there is a bowel overload.

The *kidneys*, faced with having to remove an extra load of liquid wastes or poisons from the blood stream, day after day and month after month, may enlarge. Frequency of urination increases. There is an offensive urine odour. The overload can bring about a lowered resistance to infection.

The *skin* tries hard to do its part and the sweat and sebaceous glands work overtime. But they are not up to the task. They soon cease to function properly. In acute rheumatoid arthritis, the skin has a dry sandy feeling. There is an absence of moisture associated with healthy skin. Only the palms of the hands and the soles of the feet appear to retain their ability to perspire.

Finally, the *lungs*. These have a minute-to-minute vital function to perform. The body often calls upon the lungs to shoulder the overload of the other organs of elimination. The lungs are busy ridding the blood of carbon dioxide and renewing it with oxygen for every cell in the body. Yet when the lungs must take over part of the bowel job the breath becomes fetid, unpleasant, and no mouth wash, no matter what it is called, can correct this obnoxious odour – only adequate bowel elimination can stop it.

So let's get back to where the trouble started – in the bowels.

## A 24-hour test for poison elimination

"I'm not constipated," you say. Your bowels move every day, you insist.

I am reminded of the car wash outfit that put up a big sign, "A CAR WASHED EVERY 3 MINUTES." Everybody thought that meant quick service. But when they stood waiting for their cars, yes, a car exited from the production line every three minutes but it took over 15 minutes including waiting time to have your car washed.

The daily bowel movement is fine. Two are even finer. But how long has this faecal matter resided in the intestines and bowels before elimination?

Following is a simple test *that every arthritic should make*.

At the end of one evening meal take six charcoal tablets. These are harmless. They colour your stool black. In other words, you can measure the time it takes for these to exit from your system.

The entire black should be eliminated the following morning. That is, no more black stool 12 to 14 hours after you swallowed the charcoal pills.

Usually this will not occur for arthritics. Even if they have an evacuation once or twice a day the charcoal will take up to four days and sometimes even a week to disappear.

Now when the charcoal does not disappear within 14 hours, you need help. Some laxative should be used in the evening before retiring. Your health-food store will have a selection of the best. You'll have to experiment.

The goal, you know, is that the charcoal markers must be out within 14 hours. The next night instead of charcoal eat one or two ears of corn for dinner. Do not chew some of the kernels, let them slide down whole. Undigested kernels of corn are easily noticed in the stool. The following day these should be completely eliminated.

If not, you're in hot water. The 'hot water' I mean is the enema.

Remember the enema? It was recommended by the family doctor and administered by mother to help clean out the ailing child. It was not pleasant. In fact, it was downright unpleasant. Nevertheless, it need not be as bad as the memory of it. Later I will give you some techniques to make this rather awkward procedure more acceptable.

Now, don't get me wrong. It's not going to be pleasant – despite what I read in the slick magazines (it appears that enemas are "well established" as part of sophisticated sex routines). I'm not talking about sexual gratification. I'm talking about arthritis therapy.

If the charcoal was not thoroughly eliminated in less than 14 hours, take an enema. But, to start with, use a good natural laxative.

There are many aids or laxatives on the market that you can use. I recommend them only as a temporary measure, however. Bulk fruits are your best aids to overcome constipation.

I'll tell you just what fruits to eat for your particular case in a chapter ahead. You will be doing the charcoal and corn test again to check your progress and to vary your fruit diet.*

Meanwhile, if you need instructions on how to take your first enema, turn to page 48.

## Which treatment would you rather have?

"There are so many techniques that can be used in the treatment of rheumatoid arthritis that it would take a large book to describe them all." So states the Arthritis Foundation in one of its brochures.

The postscript might be added – "and none of them successful."

Here are the ingredients of treatment mentioned: proper rest, exercise, supportive treatment, salicylates (aspirin), selected drugs, corrective surgery.

* Enemas, or colonic irrigation, should be used with caution and in moderation as they can damage delicate tissues and cause an imbalance of the body's chemicals.

## The case of Mrs M. S.

Let Mrs M. S. tell you of her experience. She is just one of millions whose stories are similar:

"I am 65 years of age and was an active business woman, always on the go until three years ago when I was finally forced to retire, due to arthritis.

"It started in 1964 when I was suddenly stricken with a very painful attack in my knees. Practically over night I found myself almost a cripple, unable to walk without pain.

"I went to a medical doctor and much to my surprise he said I had arthritis. His best advice was to take aspirin and learn to live with the condition.

"After a time, much discouraged, I went to another doctor. He showed more interest and tried everything at his command to help me – weekly gold injections, tenderil, butazolidin, and other cortisone drugs, but nothing seemed to help. I kept getting continuously worse and by this time I had to be pulled up from a chair, be helped at every step, and endured constant pain, day and night. At this point I had to completely retire from business.

"The doctor then sent me to a bone specialist who recommended an operation upon my knees. I did not want to go through this, so just continued going to the medical doctor, taking aspirin, prednisone, and B complex injections once a week, but still no relief.

"About two years ago a neighbour, who knew of Dr Campbell suggested I try him. An appointment was made. After Dr Campbell examined my knees, which by now were badly bent and swollen, making it very difficult to stand up, even for a short time, he said he believed he could help me but I would have to cooperate with him to the fullest extent. This was the first spark of hope I had been given in five years and I was most willing to faithfully follow through with any instructions.

"He told me of the natural food diet to follow and necessary treatments I needed.

"I am making a good recovery. I am now able to stand up straight, move about without pain, get a good night's sleep, do some of my housework myself, and am beginning to enjoy life again."

*Make your choice.* Which treatment would you rather have? Select A or B below:

| A | B |
|---|---|
| Rest | Special diet |
| Exercise | Aids to elimination |
| Supportive treatment | Osteopathic manipulation |
| Salicylates (aspirin) | Neuromuscular stimulation |
| Selected drugs | Selected herbs and supplements |
| Corrective surgery | Gentle and simple body-motion routines |

Perhaps there is not much difference, you say. So of course, you base your decision on which works the fastest.

You recognize A as the standard medical treatment. So maybe you choose A. And you begin.

## Treatment under plan A

*Rest.* Doctors make a serious effort to keep you from aggravating an inflamed joint by too much activity. They also try to balance rest with enough activity to keep joints mobile. You'll be resting your whole body in bed part of the time, and resting affected joints, maybe with splints, for part of the time.

*Exercise.* Doctors know how your stiffness and pain can grow with overnight immobility. So they will prescribe exercises.

*Supportive treatment.* This can mean a number of things. Doctors often prescribe hot packs, hot baths, or heat lamps. Hospitals and clinics offer hydrotherapy. Anything that warms the joints is considered helpful. Frequently a home treatment of hot paraffin wax is prescribed, where an elbow or hand is dipped into the melted wax as therapy.

*Salicylates.* Aspirin, buffered aspirin, coated aspirin, fast-dissolving aspirin, slow-dissolving aspirin. Sometimes as often as 12 times a day.

*Selected drugs.* The selection includes gold compounds, cortisone and related steroids, antimalarials, and a number of anti-inflammatory drugs.

*Corrective surgery.* Orthopaedic operations on joints are conducted to relieve pain and improve overall function. Surgery can also remove some deformities.

That is treatment A.

What is the medical *prognosis*? ..."The person with rheumatoid arthritis can be sure that better treatment will be available as the years go by," say the medical 'experts.'

If you have chosen treatment A, you are not alone. Almost all of the 13 million who now have arthritis have chosen it. They stay on treatment A year in and year out!

## Treatment under plan B

Is treatment B worth a try? You may not have to be on it more than a few weeks. Let's look at its steps.

*Special diet.* You begin largely on raw fresh fruits and vegetables and gradually add foods in a few days as your arthritis diminishes.

*Aids to elimination.* Daily enemas are advised until the raw fruits provide the necessary encouragement to keep the bowels current. Hot baths improve elimination by perspiration.

*Osteopathic manipulation.* This might be needed especially in severe cases to increase circulation – both arterial supply and venous drainage – and to initiate repair of the affected parts.

*Neuromuscular stimulation.* These are electronic vibrators that contract muscles passively and permit them to relax in a natural manner. These are available for home use and are useful, *but not mandatory*, to speed recovery. The special manual techniques of massage used by naturopaths and some osteopaths also come into this category. They help to release stiffened and thickened muscles, tendons, and ligaments.

*Selected herbs.* Dosage of aspirin or other drugs, are cut down gradually and replaced by herbs and nutritional supplements. Steroids, such as Prednisone, may need reducing much more gradually, perhaps with professional guidance. As your body takes over its own healing with the help of herbs and extra nutrients it will depend less on suppressive drugs.

*Gentle motion routines.* A vital part of the programme but never to the point of pain or fatigue.

That is treatment B.

What is the treatment B *prognosis*? ... "It is such a blessing to be free of arthritis and able to enjoy life again." The patient says it best.

What is the major difference between these two treatments, A and B? You might say the diet. Somebody else might say the manipulation.

Take another look.

The major difference is in the prognosis.

Treatment A promises relief and improvement *but treatment may have to continue indefinitely or until some new techniques are discovered*. Patients "respond well" but they are not *cured*.

Treatment B promises relief and improvement, too. But it also promises an end to the condition. Patients are cured.

Is there really any choice?

## How diet works its miracle

A man has crippling rheumatoid arthritis in both knees. His doctor recommends that the upper two wisdom teeth be removed. The extraction is performed. The teeth are removed. The arthritis remains.

A woman's husband is killed in an accident. Shortly after the tragedy, she develops painful rheumatoid arthritis in her right arm. Advised that there may be a link between the two events, she seeks psychiatric help. The emotional stress of the patient is alleviated. There even appears to be an improvement in the arthritis condition. But years later she still has painful arthritis.

A woman goes through menopause. Shortly thereafter she can no longer continue her work as a typist due to the severe pains and crippling effect of osteoarthritis. Prescribed rest and exercises are diligently followed. But the arthritis remains.

What causes rheumatoid arthritis? What causes osteoarthritis?

The answer is obviously not an infection in the teeth, tonsils, or other focal points of infection. Remove the suspected points of infection and the arthritis still remains!

The answer is obviously not stress – emotional or physical, because when the stresses are lessened or ended, the arthritis remains.

Infection, emotional stress, physical stress – all may set the climate for arthritis; *but they are not the cause.*

They merely reduce the body's ability to cope with the real cause either by adding to the total poison and waste matter to be eliminated, or by interfering with the body's restorative powers.

*What is the real cause?*

Bad nutrition!

Bad nutrition two ways:

1 A scarcity of the nutrients our body needs.
2 An overabundance of chemical additives used in the processing of foods which our body does not need and which indeed it cannot cope with.

Diet turns the trick when it is designed to correct bad nutrition. It must correct it two ways:

1 It must supply an abundance, even an overabundance, of the nutrients the body needs.
2 It must reduce, even cut off entirely, the intake of chemical additives in processed food.

This diet is the main factor in the cure of arthritis. You might experience a cure without doing another blessed thing.

You are not likely ever to experience a cure without it.

## Are you committing slow suicide?

Arthritis has no monopoly on the effects of 'civilized' nutrition. The nutrition has a strong following of killers.

If a sampling of 100 persons 20 years of age or over were to be examined for incipient arteriosclerosis, for obesity, for tuberculosis, for intestinal defects, for anaemia, and for about 15 other physical problems, fewer than 10 would pass with flying colours.

The other 90 out of 100 people would be found to have physical problems that need only further development or the right moment of stress or weakened resistance to manifest openly, and perhaps critically or chronically.

'Civilized' nutrition includes built-in self-destruction.

We are indeed committing slow suicide.

Remember when ice cream was made from the top of the whole milk and the family took turns grinding the handle of the primitive ice-cream maker?

Today it's much easier. We open a package in the freezer. We see ice cream. We taste ice cream. No labour and sweat. But what we don't see is that we are not eating a nutritious whole dairy product. We are eating what is made largely from sawdust and wood shavings.

Empty calories. With enough preservatives and artificial additives for colour and flavour to make the net nutritive value to the body – negative.

"My grandfather is 92. He smokes, drinks, and eats anything." How often do we hear that one.

I know people who can swim under water three-times longer than most, and come up smiling. I know people who can work many more hours per day than others can, and not feel it. I know people who can eat healthy, rich dinners at restaurant after restaurant week in and week out and never have a pang of indigestion.

Some of us have greater physical stamina than others. Some of us have a greater tolerance for poisons than do others. Some of us even have larger arteries and veins than others, permitting better circulation.

Let's face it. Some of us can take the gaff longer. The rest of us had better stop taking it if we want to live our life in good health.

"I am convinced that food additives are far safer in actual use than the basic natural foods ..." Who said this? It was quoted in *Life* magazine in March of 1970. It is attributed to Dr Frederick Stare, Harvard professor; the man who attacked Rachel Carson's *Silent Spring* as "propaganda."

Recently in Malaysia it was decided to use DDT in the swamps and forests to kill off malaria-carrying mosquitoes. The mosquitoes died. They were eaten by cockroaches. The cockroaches, made ill by the DDT in the mosquitoes, were caught easily and eaten by lizards. These became in turn easy prey for cats. The cats died of DDT poisoning. Rats multiplied. The fleas on rats multiplied. Bubonic plague broke out. More people were killed by plague than would have died of malaria for years.

In a way, you who have arthritis might be called lucky. You are afflicted with suffering, not death. But there is no guarantee that your suffering body, were you to continue to expose it to the slow contamination we call civilized nutrition, will not develop one or more of the more lethal imbalances or diseases.

Somebody once criticized the arthritis cure you are now learning as "merely the shotgun method." The inference was that this was not aimed at arthritis alone but was instead a sort of cure-all.

Well, then, so be it. If in the process of curing your arthritis you drop a few other ailments, will you protest?

If in the process of ridding yourself once and for all of the painful, crippling effects of arthritis, you also happen to attain a better state of general health than you have enjoyed in a long, long time, will you complain?

I know plenty of physical problems that have not been helped by this arthritis cure. Not one of these problems was arthritis itself! Except in the cases of excessive drug and gold treatments outlined in chapter 1, it has always responded.

## Poor nutrition disturbs metabolism

Every person suffering from arthritis has been found to have an imbalance in calcium and phosphorous metabolism. This is brought about either by the lack of proper intake of these basic minerals or by the lack of substances needed for their utilization. These are vitamins A and D, and the essential unsaturated fatty acids.

Now this does not mean that every person with these nutritional deficiencies will have arthritis. Some may not, due to other physical strength factors. But, I repeat, if you have arthritis, you have these deficiencies.

The vast majority of those who have suffered with arthritis for 10 years or more do not have their own teeth. Also, osteoporosis, or demineralization of the bones, is due to lack of calcium and phosphorus or the inability to use them. It is characteristic of those with arthritis.

The blood stream needs 9 milligrams of calcium per 100 cubic centimetres of volume for us to survive. To hold this level, we must supply one-seventh of an ounce daily. If we don't the body has to make up the difference by robbing the teeth and bones to support life itself.

Don't listen to those who will condemn the switch from processed to natural foods. Don't listen to cries of "food faddist." Don't be discouraged by put-down shrugs no matter how professional the shoulders.

Mankind has always resisted change. Many great scientists and thinkers of the past who dared to threaten the status quo were put in jail or otherwise prosecuted.

Around 1840, Dr Philip Semmelweiss, an Austrian physician who was associate professor of obstetrics at the University of Vienna, issued a decree: All medical students who had just been involved in dissecting corpses must first wash their hands in bichloride of mercury, a strong antiseptic, before they could examine a woman in labour.

Right across the street from the University of Vienna, where the midwives had a building, the maternity mortality was very much lower than at the University, by some 60 per cent. So, Dr Semmelweiss reasoned that the University's high rate must be related to the cadavers.

His superior; the professor of obstetrics, became so incensed with the 'heresy' of Dr Semmelweiss, that he organized enough vehement opposition to have him stoned out of Vienna. They ultimately arranged to have Dr Semmelweiss committed to an insane asylum, where he was forced to remain the rest of his life.

Health is big business. Food is big business. Anybody who rocks either boat is likely to land in trouble himself. There is many a Dr Semmelweiss nursing his wounds in this country today while people are being 'shielded' from their discoveries.

Hopefully, we will soon round the corner. As the very breath we breathe is threatened, business and industry are being brought up sharp to the realization that profit must now become subservient to the public good.

## Sixteen poisons that contribute to your arthritis

I am now going to put the finger on the poisons that one day will be prohibited from the kind of usage they now receive. It has taken years to recognize the dangers of cyclamates. After years, too, we are only on the threshold of recognizing the dangers of monosodium glutamate.

A number of additives may cause problems with arthritis. You'll find them identified on the labels of the food you buy. They are:

1 BHA (E320)
2 BHT (E321)
3 Disodium dihydrogen diphosphatase (E45Oa)
4 Monosodium glutamate (621)
5 Carageenan (E407)
6 Synthetic food colours or azo dyes
7 Sodium nitrate (E251)
8 Sodium nitrite (E250)
9 Polysorbate 60 (435)
10 Polysorbate 80 (433)
11 Di-Potassium phosphate (E340b)
12 Sorbitan-monostearate (491)
13 Oxygen interceptor
14 Sulphur dioxide (E220)
15 Sodium benzoate (E211)
16 Aluminium sodium silicate (554)

The list is actually much longer. As you read this someone is no doubt advancing yet another bright idea to make an inferior food taste better and look better. If it kills you slowly, it's all right.

- One of the newest is putting stilbeostrol in farm animals to fatten them quicker. Little matter what it does to human reproductive organs.
- Or this kind of an idea: using sulphur-dioxide gas as a stabilizer agent in the bottling of lemon juice. It works on the juice and it works on you, – slowly.
- Or this kind of an idea: putting monoglyceride in bread as an emulsifier. "I've eaten the bread for a week now with no ill effects," says the chemist. How about ten years of it?

You are now paying the price. There is inflation of a kind here, too. The price can go up. It could include heart disease, cancer, stroke, hardening of the arteries, diabetes, and more.

- Wouldn't you rather have some strawberries and cream and an order of sautéed veal kidneys for breakfast instead of that packaged dry cereal?
- Wouldn't you rather have a rare hamburger steak with a raw vegetable salad for lunch instead of that canned luncheon meat?
- Wouldn't you rather have broiled fish and fresh brussels sprouts with fresh fruit for dessert come dinner, instead of …

I'm sure you get the message by now.

## For your action

Know the sources of poisons that pollute the body and cause arthritis and other diseases as set out in this book. Banish them from your kitchen. Re-arrange your kitchen to accommodate the fresh foods that you will now enjoy. Give yourself the charcoal test, then the corn test to check on adequate elimination which is necessary to cure your arthritis.

# CHAPTER 3

# The Seven-day Programme to End Arthritic Pain and Regain Normal Use of Joints

Now you can begin your treatment. Your body will love it. Your habit department will not. If you have been suffering from arthritis, this chapter leads you through seven of the most important days of your life.

Can you imagine such acute pain from arthritis that the bed-sheets are unbearable?

Hoops had to be provided for Mrs G. W. so that the bed clothes didn't touch her pain-racked body. For six months this 42-year-old housewife had been bedridden, the culmination of six years of steadily worsening arthritis of all joints – including her jaw.

I started her immediately on the seven-day programme you are now about to receive. In two days the hoops were removed.

Let me emphasize that this patient received no medication. Her response was so dramatic that even palliation or relief with aspirin was not needed.

In seven days, all pain was gone. She was still not able to hold a cup in her hand or to turn a tap on or off. In two weeks she was walking – out of bed and doing things around the house. In three weeks cups and taps were easily handled by her. If you saw her six months later you would see no evidence that she ever had arthritis.

But we are getting ahead of ourselves.

Today is the first day of the rest of your life. A very important day. A turning point of great significance.

## The hardest day, but the only way

This seven-day programme is prescribed for both types of arthritis – either osteoarthritis or rheumatoid arthritis. The first day of this programme, the hardest of all for some, is an absolute necessity for all arthritis sufferers.

It may *not* be skipped. If you want to get the best results from the rest of the programme, make up your mind that you will persevere and be totally conscientious about adhering to its rigid requirement.

The only possible exceptions are those who are newcomers to the bursitis scene or just starting out with its playmates: tendonitis or myositis. You may skip day one.

*What happens this first day?*

*On this day you fast.*

You can begin right now as you read these lines. No need to have anything else to eat first. Start where you are. Start now!

Look at your watch. Whatever time it is now is the time you start. Tomorrow at the same time is the beginning of day number two. Then you can break your fast.

Fasting is recognized as great therapy for the body. Some people fast for five, ten, even 20 days and never miss a day at work. They feel great. They feel no hunger pangs after the first day or two. When they end their fast they feel like a new person.

Tomorrow you eat again.

Today you eat nothing.

No coffee, no tea, no soft drinks, not even fruit juices.

Water? Yes, you may drink all the water you desire. In fact, I insist that you drink at least four 8-ounce glasses of water.

Water puts no burden on your digestive or metabolic organs but it does cleanse and purify.

You will feel hunger pangs. I'll tell you just when you will feel them: your usual breakfast time, your usual lunch time, and your usual dinner time. Maybe also your usual snack time whether mid-morning or midnight.

Do these pangs mean you are hungry and in need of food? Absolutely not. They are your subconscious mind's way of reminding you it's 'time to eat.'

'Time to eat' and in need of food are two very different things.

We condition ourselves to eat by the clock. We may not salivate like Pavlov's dogs did when he rang a bell, but when the clock strikes 'meal time' there are reflexes that take place. The stomach gears itself for the food that it is conditioned to expect. We interpret these as hunger pangs.

Far from it. Your body organs are not clamouring for more work any more than you are. They are delighted to have a vacation. It's probably the first 24-hour vacation they have had for years. It will give them a chance to begin to cleanse and repair themselves.

Every part of your body will benefit. All the blood circulation and body energy utilizing in the digestive process can now go to the regenerating process. You will feel the difference. Maybe not an hour from now. But 24 hours from now you will feel as if a load has been lifted from you.

So take those protests of the body in your stride. Ignore any hunger pangs, giddiness, hunger headache. These are just automatic, thoughtless, reactions of the body due to prior programming of your subconscious computer.

Shrug them off.

Read a book.

Have a glass of water.

Tap water in some parts of the country may be quite high in nitrites and other chemicals which have seeped into water supplies from artificial fertilizers applied to agricultural land. Bottled mineral water would be preferable for your fast.

## Enjoy your vacation from food

Paul C. Bragg, the famous physical culture specialist, ran a health resort in California for over 25 years, where people came from all over the world to lose weight. Did he put them on a crash diet? No. He put them on a fast. He changed their way of eating, but the fast was the secret of his success. Some fasted seven to ten days. Just about everybody fasted one or two 24-hour periods a week.

A 24-hour fast goes swiftly. Actually, you fast every day for 12 hours; from after dinner, say 7:30 P.M. to before breakfast, 7:30 A.M. So, this is only 12 hours more.

The idea is not to count the hours or to watch the clock. Forget about food this day. Think about all the activities you will be able to enjoy once more.

Make plans for your arthritis-free life ahead.

## Set the mental climate for a physical 'miracle'

Medical records are pain-packed with case histories of arthritis setting in following a crisis in life or acute mental strain. For example:

A mother loses two sons in the war.
A father of eight loses his job.
A young woman is in a traffic accident.

In these cases there is no apparent connection between the event that appears to be the cause and the arthritis that appears to be the effect. Even in the third instance mentioned, the injuries suffered in the accident may bear no relation to the joints of the fingers where the arthritis appears.

There is no doubt that arthritis and emotions affect the body. The person who does not subject his body to the drain of negative attitudes and the stress of churning emotions has a body that is more able to cope with the physical contaminants and challenges.

*"Wait a minute, doctor. That does not apply to me. Arthritis hit me out of a blue sky."*

All right, I say, then it was the physical that was sufficient in your case *to swing the metabolic imbalance*. But now you have arthritis. Is this not an emotional strain? Does not the pain of arthritis cast a pall over even the healthiest of attitudes?

Emotional strain alters the body. Blood vessels can constrict, muscles tighten, glands malfunction. Circulation to the joints is inevitably and adversely affected.

So the *onset* of your arthritis may not have been induced by emotional strain but the *arthritis may cause emotional strain*. To this extent arthritis is perpetuating itself.

As you cut off the food poisons your body has been attempting to cope with, and as you begin to provide your body with the nutrients it needs, you can accelerate the transformation back to sparkling good health by setting the proper emotional climate for this change.

While you fast, you permit the body to rest and to recharge. Why not use this period to recharge your attitude, too!

Vera Peiffer, author of *Positive Thinking*,* has enabled millions of people to change their lives for the better by replacing the kind of attitudes that arthritis induces with optimism, joy, and expectation.

It is not easy for you to feel these positive emotions. After all, you still have arthritis. Perhaps you are not working. Finances are low. Others are taking time off from their enjoyments to help you and care for you. Perhaps your marriage is affected. And there's always the pain. These are very good reasons to feel sorry for yourself.

But today you can begin to see healing sunlight. You have every good reason to enjoy a new outlook on the future. The end of your arthritis is in sight.

### Some constructive attitudes for arthritis

Try these attitudes out for size:

- I no longer need to feel sorry for myself.
- I am ready to return to an active, enjoyable, pain-free life.
- I see myself once more as an effective, productive person.

These attitudes will help to relax taut muscles. Optimism instead of anxiety puts your body in a state of ease instead of dis-ease.

You invite a change for the better.

## The second day – delicious foods you can enjoy

Twenty-four hours after starting your fast you may begin to eat.

* Thorsons, 2001.

But 'to eat' now means quite another thing than 'to eat' meant to you yesterday.

You have a new awareness of what you have been putting into your system. You are guarding against making the same old mistakes over again.

Your fast has cleared the way for a new manner of nourishing, not needling, the body. You are ready for the refreshing taste of 'living' foods.

Today is a day of fresh raw fruits and fresh raw vegetables. I repeat two works for emphasis so that there can be no misunderstanding:

- Fresh
- Raw

In fruits, take your pick of fresh raw apples, pears, bananas, all types of fresh (not frozen) berries, nectarines, plums, peaches, cherries. Of course, all of these may not be available, depending on the season. Dried fruits, like raisins, prunes, figs, and dates are acceptable only if sun ripened. Read the package very carefully to make sure chemicals have not been added. Also, consider grapes and melons, all varieties.

### Citrus fruits

Do not use citrus fruits in the acute stages of arthritis. Keep away, at least for now from oranges, grapefruits, lemons, limes, kumquats, and tangerines.

### Vegetables

In vegetables, you have a selection of zesty, flavourable bounty all-year-round in most parts of the country. Some may have travelled a few days since the picking but that does not do as much harm as cooking and canning, or cooking and freezing. You are always likely to find carrots, cabbage, brussels sprouts, leeks, chives, radishes, onions, green peppers, beets, endive, watercress, and lettuce. Available for much of the year too, are green peas, string beans, wax beans, haricot beans, spinach, kohlrabi, Swiss chard, parsnips, aubergines.

Early in the growing season we get asparagus and rhubarb. Late in the growing season we get all varieties of delicious squash and we get cauliflower and winter kale.

> Buy organic products wherever possible. Modern farming methods may leave residues of insecticide and fertilizer on the fruits and vegetables available in supermarkets. Always wash all fruit and vegetables well, and peel non-organic fruit; unfortunately peeling removes some of the nutrients, but avoids further contamination of your body with unwanted chemicals.

"But how can you eat these raw?" you ask.

Have you ever tasted raw spinach? It goes into gourmet salads. Raw cauliflower is a popular cocktail party hors d'oeuvre. Raw carrots are grated into many dishes. Raw string beans disappear into many a mouth as they are being prepared in the kitchen as do peas, and other common vegetables.

Vegetables are delicious raw. What's more they are potent nutrients when raw, less so when cooked. Cooking, especially when lots of water is used, wastes the minerals and vitamins of vegetables and leaves them only a shadow of their former nutritious selves.

A more complete list of fruits and vegetables available to you – fresh and raw – appears in chapter 7.

One more food may be enjoyed today. It is one of the most nutritious, body-building foods available. That food is liver.

Here again, the idea of eating it raw may throw some people. I have found, however, they will enjoy it if just partially cooked. Try to add raw liver to your first day's regimen. If you must cook it, cook it only slightly.

> Buy organic calves liver. If this is not possible, purchase liver from a source known to use a minimal amount of agricultural chemicals. The liver has many important biological functions, one of which is de-toxification and storage of unwanted materials taken into the body. Liver from young animals is your best choice.

Here is another idea. Take fresh raw beef liver (the Kosher liver is preferable for freshness) or raw pork or lamb liver, and, using an electric blender, grind it together with a mixture of fruits and vegetables. Those who try this not only enjoy the blended meal but look forward to inventing new variations and proportions.

If you are squeamish about eating raw liver, sauté it lightly in butter or freshly rendered beef suet. Remember, it is the *raw liver* that is best for you, so cook it minimally.*

A word of caution about how you enjoy blended foods. The blender, in effect, does most of our chewing for us. As a result, we are tempted to 'drink' what comes out of the blender. We swallow it quickly without chewing. This does not give our saliva a chance to mix thoroughly with what we swallow. Saliva is important to the digestive process.

So, if you cannot get yourself to chew a semi-liquid food, at least swish it around in your mouth a few seconds before you swallow.

You may find one meal is enough this second day. Or you may break the fast with just some raw fruit, later have a raw salad, and then go on to the liver and more raw vegetables and fruit for a third meal.

Vegetarians can avoid these animal sources of protein and iron by substituting sunflower seeds, tofu (soya bean curd), soya milk and more vegetables, such as watercress and green peppers. For example, you can blend tofu with yogurt, tahini, and watercress to make a delicious dip (see recipe page 149).

## The third day – add more foods

On the third day all the food that lives under more than three-quarters of the surface of the earth is yours – seafood.

Best of all is raw untreated milk but this is almost impossible to find nowadays even if you can buy direct from the farm. Goats' or sheeps' milk may be a good alternative, especially for people who

---

* If you suffer from gout, avoid eating liver and other organ meats. See pages 190–92.

are intolerant of cows' milk. Soya milk is another good choice. Your local health-food store may be able to suggest suppliers.

Of course, fresh seafood is another story. There should always be plenty of that around in most parts of the country.

At the very top of my list are fish roe and, you may have guessed, fish liver. Then, of course, there are striped bass, shrimp, lobster, all shellfish, salmon, tuna (fresh!), halibut, cod.* Check the list in chapter 7, but it is a limited list and omissions are not intended as disallowance.

The sea is the limit – but not polluted lakes and streams. Maybe even some day we will not be able to trust seafood. Meanwhile, Bon Appetit for seafoods.

For those living in rural interior areas where seafood is not available, you have two alternatives:

1  You may substitute frozen seafood. These products must be
   uncooked and unprocessed. No fish cakes, or fish sticks.
   Sometimes the fish is filleted, that is, most of the bones
   removed. That is all right, but absolutely no breading or
   preparation of other sort. I'm not taking the lid off frozen
   vegetables unless they are not precooked before freezing.
2  You may substitute other organ meats. Hearts, brains,
   sweetbreads, tripe, and kidneys are all available in large meat
   markets. Try them. Check your cookbooks for best ways to
   prepare them. (There are some recipes in chapter 8.) Always
   cook these as little as possible consistent with your taste
   preference. Vegetarian alternatives to meat and fish abound.
   See the recipes chapter.

## When pain and heat disappear

Within three to ten days your pain should end and the heat and swelling in the joints should disappear.

Some doctors still say that there is no such thing as an 'arthritis diet.' Maybe this is not an 'arthritis diet.' But if it ends arthritis

---

* If you suffer from gout, avoid fish roe, shellfish, lobster, and shrimp. See page 56.

pains, if it causes the arthritis swelling and the heat in arthritic joints to subside, if it starts your recovery from arthritis, what name would you give it?

You can now begin to add new foods to your menus but first let me remind you of something you should be doing, in these first few days especially.

### Don't forget elimination

*Proper elimination is just as important as proper food intake*. If the charcoal and corn tests, described in the previous chapter, show the least delay in bowel functioning, take an enema. If you need instructions jump ahead to chapter 5 and read the step-by-step procedure for properly administering an enema to yourself.

### The case of Mrs H. G.

I am often more surprised than the patient by the speed with which recovery takes place. Mrs H. G. was bedridden most of the time, wore a brace, and was almost completely incapacitated. Yet, seven years of suffering was ended in seven days under my care.

But let her tell you in her own words:

"I had been in an auto accident which affected my spine and caused chronic arthritis. I was semi-invalid, in and out of bed, and suffered with severe pain in my upper back and left shoulder. No day was without pain and the frustration attending a crippling arthritic condition. I couldn't raise my arms without severe pain; combing my hair was almost impossible. I could not grasp a cup or a tool firmly enough to handle it. My work is sculpture and etching. I was compelled to abandon it. There were sporadic remissions but only of short duration.

"Doctors gave me up to 24 aspirins per day, sleeping pills, tranquillizers and opiates over a period of seven years. In addition, I was given traction, hydrotherapy, sonic-ray therapy, and physiotherapy, and wore neck braces regularly. I spent time at a fine hospital under the care of the chief, but with little relief.

"I continued without improvement in spite of prolonged bed rest. Unrelated surgery had forced me into complete rest and inactivity which was my last hope for relief from the constant pain. While I was *completely* inactive I found relief. As soon as I started normal activity I was again in severe pain. I seemed to be faced with the impossible choice between invalided inactivity or unbearable pain.

"It was at this time I began treatment with Dr Campbell. I was at my worst and dejected because I could not continue my work. After treatment started, I felt a tremendous improvement in seven days. Within two weeks the brace was off and I felt better in a gradual movement constantly upward. It was like a miracle that I could begin driving, lift things, commence working again. My whole outlook changed and it gave me courage to do what I thought would be impossible, everything. I took a trip abroad three months after starting the treatment and was able to sit in a car for two to three hours at a time. Previous to this I had to lie down on the back seat because the jogging motion of the car caused too much pain.

"I am now lifting heavy things in my sculpture work, raising my arms for long periods, driving one hour each way to a nearby city. In short, I have become a complete human being. I do not have pain and take no medication at all. I am sleeping well and have found beauty and harmony in living again."

Let me repeat – diet and elimination are necessary to control your arthritis.

Where the disease is of long standing then you might also need osteopathic manipulation and neuromuscular stimulation to hasten joint recovery – that is, the restoration of bone structure. More about these aids in later chapters.

### Introducing a variety of foods

Meanwhile, you can begin to add a variety of foods to your diet.

First, you may add cheese. You may choose natural cheese as opposed to processed cheese. Look at the packages carefully. It is either 'processed' or 'natural.' Select the 'natural'; be sure it is made of whole milk, either whole goats', sheep, or cows' milk. Do not use even 'natural' cheese made from skimmed milk.

In the days ahead – one food at a time – you can add meats such as chops, steaks, and roasts. Undercooked is preferred. Learn to appreciate meat rare, almost raw.

> Do not be tempted to buy ground or minced meat. Make your own, using the leanest, best-quality meat you can afford. Many times ground meat is just what you need to make a favourite meal, but all commercially processed meat is open to contamination by rapidly growing bacteria.

The chops can be either pork, lamb, or veal. Steaks are fine whether beef, venison, ham, or lamb. Turkey, duck, and geese are permitted. Geese are especially desirable since their dark meat, from grass feeding, contains more amino acids and is therefore more nutritious. As to chicken, those that are free-range, fed out in the open, are fine. I would avoid the usual poultry farm product where the fowl seldom see the sun and never peck in the fields but instead eat only prepared feed. These are not natural chickens. Some commercially raised chickens even have arthritis themselves.

> Many people think that free-range poultry always tastes best. Buy birds that are reared using organic methods. The meat has better texture, and is more likely to contain more nutrients your body needs.

A word of caution here is needed. Sometimes, when meat is added, increased stiffness may be noticed the next morning. If so, discontinue the meat for a week and then try it again. If stiffness does not return, it can be added regularly to the diet. If stiffness recurs, discontinue the meat for two weeks and then try again. This time, stiffness most likely will not occur.

Observe yourself carefully each time you add a new food to the diet. Remember, only one new food should be added at a time, to determine whether or not it causes joint stiffness the next day. Rarely will joint pain return. If it does, that food should, of course, be eliminated. Note it on your 'culprit' list of foods to be avoided.

As your arthritis condition improves, other natural foods may be added one at a time. Be sure to include fresh nuts. Then add cooked vegetables, such as cauliflower, rutabagas, squash, kale, broccoli, parsnips, and Swiss chard. Use a minimum of water and then *undercook*.

## Cheating on yourself – you may get away with it

A patient was so overjoyed with his rapid recovery he had a large order of french fries with his steak. He called me the next day. "Doc," he confided, "I cheated last night." He told me the gruesome details. "How long do I have to wait before the pains start?" My reply, "Maybe forever," surprised him.

Those who have had arthritis severely, over a long period of time, and who have suffered great joint deformity, should remain on this nutritional programme indefinitely.

Others with slight joint involvement and of relatively short duration (say less than a year), may cheat on their list occasionally with no harm; but you should always be on your guard for adverse symptoms or flareups

If and when these flareups occur, you must immediately revert back to the straight and narrow path. You must go back to the original week's starter diet.

If you follow this treatment schedule, there should be no joint pain flareup at all. Some have an aggravation of symptoms when the weather changes, due to, in large measure, a change in atmospheric pressure. As time goes on you will find it gratifying to see that weather changes become less and less bothersome. In fact, at the end of six months weather changes usually have no effect at all, providing you have been eating as advised.

## *The oil that hastens recovery*

The food you are enjoying this first week of basic treatment is rich in nutrients. But not rich enough.

Your body needs more natural oil. It needs more vitamin A and vitamin D.

These needs spell 'cod liver oil.'

I advise all who suffer from arthritis to begin to take one table-spoon of cod liver oil twice daily beginning with the second day. Since the taste of this marvellous nutrient leaves much to be desired, try the cod liver oil capsules.

Do not take daily any more cod liver oil or cod liver oil capsules than are necessary to supply 10,000 International Units (IU) of vitamin A, or 1,000 IU of vitamin D. Read the label on the bottle or ask the manager of your health-food store or chemist. Then adjust your dosage accordingly.

Cod liver oil has been recognized for its value to arthritis sufferers for the last 50 years or more. Writing in the Archives of Internal Medicine in March, 1920, Dr Ralph Pemberton told of the improvement experienced by most of 400 soldier patients to whom he gave cod liver oil.*

But cod liver oil needs no defence. It has been dispensed by doctors for decades to combat vitamin D deficiency, especially when evidenced in the bones by such symptoms as rickets, curvature of the spine and retarded growth.

Cod liver oil helps cure arthritis.

## *"But, Doctor, I'm not allowed to eat that"*

The diet I have given you will play a major role in controlling your arthritis. It is the key factor. Yet there are many who say, "I can't eat these things because of my ..." And they point to their ulcers or gall bladder or colitis condition or other ailment.

---

* The inflammation of arthritis is reduced by the action of nutrients known as omega-3 fatty acids. These are found in cod liver oil, but are more highly concentrated in pure fish oil. For more information about why fish oil is a better choice than cod liver oil, see page 139.

I say these foods will not hurt specific ailments but will instead help them to correct themselves in the long run. But if you have any concern, then shift over gradually.

Fast the first day. Eat what you can of the arthritis diet the second day, converting over fully as you prove to yourself that it helps, not hurts.

It has to help. The natural foods supply the intestinal muscle fibres and, indeed, the muscle fibres of all of your vital organs with the nutrients they need to function properly.

### Ulcers

Ulcers* are often induced by worry and in your case you may be removing the very cause of that worry when you get rid of your arthritis and are able to move around again. But meanwhile, the physical handmaiden of ulcers is constipation. Constipation will disappear when you banish artificial, devitalized, demineralized foods from your diet and substitute nature's bountiful nutrients.

If you are concerned about the effect of raw fruit or vegetables on your ulcer try mixing them in a blender or serving them lightly cooked or steamed.

### Gall bladder

Gall bladders need nutrients to function properly, too. Can you imagine a gall bladder that functions on liquor, beer, coffee, sugar, coke, ice cream, spaghetti, pizza, and chocolate layer cake – yet won't function on crisp salads, fresh fruits, and other natural foods? It just cannot fail to function on natural foods.

### Colitis

And what about colitis? Here there is a factor that dictates a slow transition period. Mucous colitis can expose sensitive membranes to irritation. Raw fruits and raw vegetables should be put on hold for a week or two. Stay with the fresh seafood, animal organ meats, and the cod liver oil. Then gradually move onto the raw

---

* If you have ulcers, avoid using aspirin and ibuprofen for pain control, as they both may cause gastric upset. See pages 105–107 for more information.

fruits, especially bananas, and cooked vegetables, then slightly cooked, then raw. You should, however, continue your *bowel markers* – *charcoal* tablets. This is essential. It is a must. Food waste from one evening meal must be eliminated within 14 hours.

There are one or two other supplements to the diet that everybody will find valuable.

## Brewers' yeast – an essential supplement

Besides cod liver oil, there are some other food supplements that are brimming with what your body is aching for.

It is said that more nutrients are concentrated in *brewers' yeast* than in any other food known to man. Some day brewers' yeast may be the answer to the undernourishment of an overpopulated world. It needs little soil, yet provides rich food value.

Yeast is a vegetable micro organism that is rich in protein. It contains hardly any sugar or starch and, in fact, breaks down sugar. It is not exactly palatable, but there are a number of varieties in health-food stores that cater to the taste buds.

Remember we are talking about *brewers' yeast* not bakers' yeast. *Bakers' yeast can even be dangerous to take.* Brewers' yeast is a different story. Brewers' yeast is excellent for you. If you cannot find it easily, try the health-food store.

Brewers' yeast is just about the least expensive protein you can buy. It is also one of the best sources of the important family of B vitamins. The science of nutrition is discovering more and more about how the body depends on B vitamins. Another excellent source is liver.

I recommend that you put one tablespoon of powdered brewers' yeast into your 8-ounce glass of raw certified milk once a day.

I also recommend that you add one tablespoon of *blackstrap molasses* to that milk drink. It is one of the richest sources of body-usable iron. It is also rich in other needed minerals, such as phosphorus, and in some of the B vitamins. It makes a healthy sweetening.

## The myth about drinking lots of water

Future doctors are being taught in many medical schools that a person should drink six to eight 8-ounce glasses of water per day depending on his weight – one glass per 20 pounds. The source for this precept is undisclosed but it is perpetuated from medical teacher to student.

In some cases the admonition of doctor to patient to drink all this water "to keep the system clean and to flush the kidneys" sinks into the subconscious. Then nature's call for water – that familiar thirsty feeling – is ignored in favour of the doctor's instructions.

Actually our body does not need such large quantities of water especially when we eat fruits and vegetables, and when we drink two or three glasses of milk a day. We can trust nature's call for water just as faithfully as we can trust her call for us to get rid of urine.

We should drink only when we are thirsty.

I have occasionally come across people who were water addicts. A water addict usually starts the morning with eight to ten glasses of water. It gives them a feeling of well-being or intoxication. As the feeling wears off, they take another glass or two. It helps them to keep the 'glow' on. Some 18 or 20 glasses later, they go to bed still in an intoxicated state.*

Too much water places a load on the kidneys. When the kidneys cannot handle it, the excess water backs up into other parts of the system including the blood. Watery blood means lower body efficiency and lessened mental activity.

Drink only when you are thirsty. Don't look upon water as the all-purifying liquid you need. It may be just the opposite.

The days of really pure water are numbered. Water supplies are becoming progressively more contaminated. And as fast as this happens, man must tamper more and more with the water, adding

---

* Drinking between $1^1/2$ and 2 litres of water a day helps maintain a healthy body; the higher amount needed if you participate in demanding physical activity, consume large quantities of protein, or suffer from bouts of cystitis. Drinking water will not make you fat, as some people seem to think. It is a vital part of internal cleaning.

bacteria-killing chemicals and other substances. Net result: water may soon be as much an 'impurifier' as it has been thought to be a purifier.

Dr Campbell's prophetic statement about water quality demonstrates how much in tune he was with the link between our environment and how we live. In urban areas, the tap water we drink has been recycled many times, and although it meets the strict standards set by health officials, it remains contaminated with chemicals that are not natural parts of the human body. Bottled waters from well-known sources are less likely to contain unwanted chemical residues. Filtering your tap water gives a better-tasting product with fewer chemical residues. Buy the best-quality water filter you can afford.

## Foods that must never be eaten again

Steak, you can eat. Eggs, yes. Cheese, yes. Potatoes, yes. Add them to your diet. You can add food after food to your permanent arthritis-free life.

Those who are newcomers to the crippling effects of arthritis can add foods faster than those who must permit their joints to rehabilitate themselves from long-term effects.

But nobody – I repeat, nobody – should ever return to the hardcore troublemakers that I have already warned you about.

I am repeating a list of these so there can be no mistake.

These are no-no all the way.

Avoid them altogether – today and tomorrow. The more you adhere to this strict prohibition, the more healthful tomorrows you will have.

## The foods that should be permanently avoided:

- Flour of all kinds, whether it is whole wheat (unless grown without artificial fertilizers and poisonous sprays), white flour, corn flour, rye flour, soy flour, etc.

- All flour products like bread, toasts, cakes, pies, cookies, crackers, buns, doughnuts, spaghetti, macaroni, noodles, pizza, etc.
- Coffee, tea, cocoa, liquor, beer, wine, colas, carbonated beverages and all so-called "soft drinks."
- Sugars, candies, ice cream, and artificial sweeteners. Jellies, jams, and marmalades.
- Canned or processed foods, such as custards, puddings, and prepared mixes.
- Frozen fruits.
- Any food manufactured or adulterated by man, such as prepared breakfast cereals or semi-prepared ones like quick-cooking oatmeal.

Dr Campbell's arthritis programme calls for the elimination of all processed foods from your diet, and that includes all products made with wheat flour. Many people find their arthritis pain improves very soon after eliminating wheat from their diet. This is probably because they are sensitive to the gluten in wheat. For more information about gluten, see pages 210 and 211. Other grains containing gluten are rye, barley, and oats. Try to eliminate these grains – in all forms – from your diet.

I can hear the cries of protest all the way across the country. "What is there left to eat?"

It's an old story. I see jaws drop when I hand patients this list. Then a few weeks later they are all smiles.

It's just as easy to break the bread and cereal habit as it was to create it. It's just as easy to forget about coffee and tea as it was to refrain from these beverages in your childhood days.

### A helpful technique

Let me give you a reinforcing technique right here and now. It is based on successful auto-conditioning methods used by over-weight people who want to make it easier for themselves to break the sweets habit.

A recent book* on this technique calls it the 'two-path' exercise. It is very effective. Here is what you can do right now to begin to break away from foods dangerous to arthritics:

1 Sit in a comfortable chair with this book opened to the list of foods to be permanently avoided.
2 Close your eyes gently after reading these instructions and visualize yourself at a fork in the road. To the left you see yourself eating the no-no foods on the list. Your life along this road is pain-racked with arthritis. To the right you see yourself eating freshly prepared foods, non-processed fresh fruits, meats, and vegetables. Your life along this path is pain-free, healthy, vigorous.
3 You see yourself taking the right-hand road to a better life.

## Seven-day menu for a new pain-free life

Now, I am going to recap the first seven days for you, so that there can be no misunderstanding. Copy the no-no list and paste it in an obvious spot in the kitchen.

Alongside it you can paste up a copy of this seven-day programme, adding 'approved' foods as you move into subsequent days and weeks in the arthritis-cure programme.

At any rate, the menu that follows is based on optimum food values and results. Substitutions are permissible (but not from the 'no' list) in accordance with availability and personal preference.

*Day 1*

| *Breakfast* | – None |
| *Lunch* | – None |
| *Dinner* | – None |
| | Drink at least four 8-ounce glasses of water (use bottled mineral or spring water if possible). |

---

\* *How to Strengthen Your Life With Mental Isometrics* by Sidney Petrie and Robert B. Stone, Parker Publishing Co., West Nyack, N.Y.

### Day 2

| | | |
|---|---|---|
| *Breakfast* | – | Unsweetened grape or prune juice. Bananas |
| *Lunch* | – | Fresh beef liver, preferably raw or lightly sautéed.* Mixed green salad, oil and cider vinegar dressing. Bowl of blackberries or other fruit in season. |
| *Dinner* | – | Raw vegetable plate (green peppers, celery, tomatoes, etc.) Raw fruit salad (shredded apples, figs, grapes, bananas, etc., but no citrus fruits) Take one tablespoon of cod liver oil, twice a day.** |

### Day 3

| | | |
|---|---|---|
| *Breakfast* | – | Blended raw fruits 8-oz raw certified milk*** |
| *Lunch* | – | Fresh fillet of ocean fish lightly sautéed. Raw cauliflower or other raw fresh vegetable.**** |

---

\*    Vegetarian alternatives to these items may be used instead. A wide variety of recipes using rice, millet, lentils, buckwheat, chickpeas, tofu, tahini, cheese, eggs, and mushrooms are permissible. NB PEOPLE WITH GOUT SHOULD ALSO AVOID LIVER AND KIDNEYS AS THEY ARE HIGH IN URIC ACID. Other foods that increase the likelihood of an attack of gout are shellfish, shrimp, and lobster.

\*\*   Many experts suggest substituting 500mg fish oil twice a day for the cod liver oil prescribed here.

\*\*\*  Some people with arthritis cannot tolerate cows' milk. Use goats' milk, sheep milk, or unsweetened soya milk as alternatives.

\*\*\*\* If you suffer from gout, avoid eating asparagus, spinach, rhubarb, peas, beans, and lentils. Celery helps eliminate uric acid, and should be included in your diet at least twice a week.

8-oz raw certified milk with 1 tbl spoon of powdered brewers' yeast and 1 tbl spoon of blackstrap molasses.***

Dinner — Fresh (or Kosher) beef liver lightly sautéed with onions.* Mixed green salads.
Melon, or other fruit in season.
8-oz raw certified milk.***
Take one tablespoon of cod liver oil, or 500mg fish oil, twice a day.**

## Day 4

Breakfast - Prunes or prune juice.
8-oz raw certified milk.***

Lunch — Veal kidneys, lightly sautéed.*
Mixed green salad.
8-oz raw certified milk with 1 tbl spoon of powdered brewers' yeast and 1 tbl spoon of blackstrap molasses.***

Dinner — Halibut steak (or other seafood) broiled.*
Raw spinach salad.
Half avocado.
Strawberries or other fruit in season.
8-oz raw certified milk.***
Take one tablespoon of cod liver oil, or 500mg fish oil, twice a day.

## Day 5

Breakfast — Melon half, or other raw fruit in season.
8-oz raw certified milk.***

Lunch — Half avocado, sliced tomatoes, and watercress.
8-oz raw certified milk with 1 tbl spoon of powdered brewers' yeast and 1 tbl spoon of blackstrap molasses.***

Dinner — Fresh beef liver patties, as rare as you can eat them.*
Mixed green salad.

Soaked, dried apricots.
8-oz raw certified milk.***
Take one tablespoon of cod liver oil, or
500mg fish oil, twice a day.

*Day 6*

*Breakfast*     – Unsweetened grape or prune juice.
Veal kidneys lightly sautéed.*
8-oz raw certified milk.***

*Lunch*     – Shrimp salad.*
Melon half, or other raw fruit in season.
8-oz raw certified milk with 1 tbl spoon of
powdered brewers' yeast and 1 tbl spoon
of blackstrap molasses.***

*Dinner*     – Large chef's salad induding raw peas, raw
string beans, and other uncooked vegeta-
bles and greens.
Plums, or other raw fruit in season.
8-oz raw certified milk.***
Take one tablespoon of cod liver oil, or
500mg fish oil, twice a day.

*Day 7*

*Breakfast*     – Sliced bananas.
8-oz raw certified milk.***

*Lunch*     – Lightly broiled fillet of sole.*
Carrot sticks and watercress.
Grapes.
8-oz raw certified milk.***

*Dinner*     – Lightly sautéed sweetbreads.*
Raw vegetables mixed in blender.
Honeydew melon or other raw fruit in
season.
8oz raw certified milk.***
Take one tablespoon of cod liver oil,
or 500mg fish oil, twice a day

## Special instructions for all seven days

1 Drink only when thirsty, and then only juice of raw fresh fruit, or juice of raw fresh vegetables, or raw certified milk, or water.
2 Take an enema daily until charcoal and corn test shows no further need. Follow instructions in chapter 5.*
3 Continue this diet until heat, pain, and swelling disappear.
4 Add one food per day after heat, pain, and swelling disappear, only from the allowable lists in chapter 7.

## For action

• Go shopping for the foods you will eat the first seven days: animal organ meats, fresh ocean fish, fresh vegetables, fresh fruits.
• Use the seven days of menus at the close of the chapter as your guide.
• Begin the seven-day programme with a one-day fast.
• Stay on the programme until pain, swelling, and heat, are ended.

* Many experts feel that enemas should be avoided unless used as a treatment of last choice in cases of constipation. The delicate tissues lining the colon are adapted to removing excess fluid from faeces, and may be damaged by excessive exposure to external fluids.

# CHAPTER 4

# How to Break Arthritis-Causing Habits Once and for All

It takes strong willpower to change eating habits. Look at all the overweight people around us who have tried willpower and failed. In this chapter you will find a substitute for willpower. Use this substitute as shown in this chapter and you will slip into your new arthritis-free eating habits quickly, easily, and without an ounce of willpower. If changing your present eating habits is like a hard-to-take medicine, then this chapter makes it all an easy-to-take capsule.

We live in a polluted world.

The air we breathe, the water we drink and swim in, the food we eat – these are all changing. The change is away from a naturally pure state to an unnatural and impure state.

Man's body is changing, too. It is responding to this different environment. It is adjusting itself. It is accommodating today more impurity than it could possibly have tolerated 50 years ago.

But the whole process is accelerating. Even the rate of acceleration is accelerating. We are rushing headlong into this toxic world faster than our body can adjust to it. The result: chronic and acute disease, premature ageing, and death before our time.

Nevertheless there is hope!

Some two years ago legislation was proposed by the US Congress to curb cosmetics that contain mercury or mercury compounds. The Federal Food and Drug Administration has recommended that mercury used as a preservative in skin lotions be replaced by a less toxic substance as it causes an appreciable hazard to persons using significant quantities of it on a regular basis. In the UK, mercuric salts are still used in a wide variety of cosmetics as a preservative, although mercury and mercury compounds are no longer used in cosmetics.

I cite this as only one instance of hundreds evidencing an increasing vigilance against new harmful toxins. Perhaps the day is not too far off when the acceleration will be slowed and man will be able to adjust to a more slowly changing environment.

Since that day is not here yet, each person must be his own protector:

- We must avoid adding new types of toxic substances to our food, water, cosmetics, clothing, air, medication, etc.
- We must break present habits that bind us to existing toxic substances.

It is not easy to break the coffee or the tea habit. Many of us have grown dependent on it. We find it comforting, stimulating, enjoyable.

It is not easy for many of us to resist a cold soft drink on a hot day, or a doughnut with that coffee, or a sandwich for lunch, or crackers with our soup, or candy, cake, and ice cream.

It may seem like the end of all fun in the world to chuck the booze. No martinis at lunch, no scotch before dinner, no wine during dinner, no beer while watching TV.

But it's the beginning, not the end. It's the beginning of new zestful days, of brimming good health, of the years rolled back to a new feeling of youthfulness.

Cigarette smokers who finally break the habit are usually ecstatic about how great they feel, that fresh feeling in their mouth ("I can taste food again"), that liberation from the weed.

It is the same when we break other health-eroding habits. We are renewed, invigorated, revitalized.

It is all well worth it.

In this chapter I am going to help you make transitions from old eating ways to new eating ways as easy as pie, only pie won't be easy any more. I am going to give you simple mental exercises that actually change your habits for you *without any willpower on your part.* In effect, you will be trading a few minutes a day of comfortable mental imaging for days and maybe weeks of broken resolutions, guilty conscience, and painful resistance to temptation of certain foods.

The psychologists use these exercises to help people break out of habit-formed prisons. They know how difficult such habits can be to break. They say, in fact, that the harder you try, the more likely you are to fail!

Here is the easy way to rid yourself of arthritis-causing habits.

## How to reprogramme your subconscious computer

When we do anything over and over again, we train ourselves to do it more easily, without conscious thinking or effort. Learning to walk, to ride a bicycle, to drive a car, to play the piano, to use a typewriter – all require a repetition, practice, before the act becomes an unconscious one, where we don't have to consciously exert ourselves any more. Then it is as easy as drinking coffee or eating cake.

If you were to substitute herb tea for coffee for several weeks, you could develop a taste for herb tea. What this really means is that you are conditioning yourself to enjoy it in place of whatever you drank habitually before. This is a process of conditioning. It is a rather long process. Like practising and learning how to drive a car, it takes time. But there is a shortcut.

You can condition yourself faster, almost overnight. It necessitates your reaching your subconscious mind and changing the instructions it now operates under.

The subconscious mind is a servomechanism. That is, it obediently regulates our behaviour according to what we programme into it. Those who are not aware of this fact are themselves the slave of their own servomechanism. They keep on behaving in ways that work against their own health and happiness. Know how to feed your mental servomechanism with the right instructions and you become the master of it and of your own destiny

It does not matter what kind of arthritis you have. The seven-day diet will banish heat, swelling, and pain – if you stay on it.

For many, that diet will be all that is necessary. No enemas, no osteopathic manipulations, no medicines, no neurological stimulation, no special exercises.

Surely the promise of quick relief and ultimate cure is reason enough to want to stay on the diet for as long as needed, and then to stay off the culprit foods – forever.

### The two-step programme

Here are two steps that enable you to reprogramme your subconscious servomechanism to keep you on the right foods, off the wrong foods, all done without willpower.

*Step one.* Learn how to relax your body and quiet your mind so that you are totally limp and tranquil.
*Step two.* See yourself eating the right foods and enjoying them, avoiding the wrong foods and being better off for it.

## Relaxation – doorway to the subconscious

Why is relaxing the body and quieting the mind necessary? Actually, you could do step two without step one and eventually you would change your behaviour. Step one hastens the results.

The reason is that it 'folds back' the conscious mind and permits your mental images to be fed more effectively into the subconscious. When the conscious mind is out of the way, it does not interfere through critical evaluation, subjective attitudes, and doubts or negativity

Relax, and your mental images are received loud and clear by the subconscious. You are reprogramming it. The results are instant!

### A powerful case history

"Parties are my downfall," said one woman in her forties who had a recurrence of severe arthritic knee pains after a year of respite from them. Of course, I immediately probed for the cause in her diet. She admitted to not knowing how to be sociable at a cocktail party without a drink in her hand. Then the drink led to hors d'oeuvres. I promised her cocktail parties without knee pains. She agreed to cooperate. Here is what she did:

*First,* she learned how to relax deeply after selecting the method that seemed most comfortable. Next, she saw herself in mental imaging sessions while relaxed having a wonderful time at parties with a drink in her hand – *water.* Finally, she used reinforcing mental images of liquor causing her pain, and water purifying her.

"I had a great time Saturday night," she reported to me two weeks later. "I was the life of the party on three ice-clinking glasses of water. Everybody thought I was drinking vodka on the rocks. They didn't realize how true it was when I told them I was feeling no pain."

Try this now: read the ten steps below. Read them again so you will know what to do without having to look at the book in the middle. Then do them.

### The basic ten steps in your mental programme

1 Sit in a comfortable chair. Wiggle your toes and adjust your feet, arms, and back to be perfectly comfortable.
2 Take three deep breaths to let go of all the tension.
3 Tense your left hand by making a fist. Then let go and feel what 'limp' really means. Do the same with your other hand, leg muscles, face muscles (force a grin then let go).
4 Enjoy a feeling of limp, relaxed heaviness creep over your entire body, until you are so relaxed you become conscious of your breathing.
5 Know that with every breath you take you go deeper and deeper into this beautiful state of total looseness, agelessness, limpness.
6 Quieten the mind. Let thoughts drift through until there are no more and your mind is like a clean slate.
7 See yourself enjoying your meals pain-free – meals of fresh green salads, raw fruits, organ meats, fresh raw vegetables. Feel the fresh crisp taste, the alive flavours. See yourself happy, healthy, and full of vibrant energy.

8  See yourself go into an even deeper state of relaxation faster next time you follow this programme.

9  Tell yourself you will emerge from this quiet state on the count of three feeling wonderful.

10 Count aloud. One, two, *three*!

You have just taken a step towards re-conditioning yourself to more healthful eating habits and an arthritis-free life.

You need to do this once or twice a day to reinforce the beneficial effects. Soon any other way of eating but the 'right' way will be unnatural and difficult for you.

The process of relaxation and visualization is more popularly known as self-hypnosis. It is safe, harmless, and effective. You do not lose consciousness or go into a trance. You merely approach a sort of sleepy wakefulness. You may stop at any time – if the doorbell or phone rings or someone enters the room. You can do it any place where you can relax.

## Effective visualization – pictures of things to come

The better and deeper you can relax, the more successful you will be. Your visualized pictures are etched deeper into the mind when you are quiet in both mind and body.

Some people find it difficult to visualize. Here is an exercise to test your ability to see a picture in your mind's eye.

Close your eyes, visualize a black dot. Now see a red circle around it. Now, put a yellow circle around the red one. Can you see all three? Then go one step further. Put a green circle around the yellow. Some will be able to add one or two more colours.

### An alternative plan

If you had trouble with that one, then here's one you'll find really easy. Close your eyes and try to recall the last time you had duck or turkey. What was the occasion? Whose home were you at? Who else was there? What did they wear? What else was on the menu? How did it taste?

The pictures we hold in our mind are the shadows of things to come. If you have been ill with arthritis so long a time that you forget what it is like to be pain-free and well, then you had better do some heavy recalling as to when you were free from arthritis.

If you cannot see yourself well, you are working against yourself. If you can see yourself full of vim and vigour and bubbling with zest, you are helping yourself to get there.

Your mind remembers everything. Just ask it. Then sit back and wait to accept what *it* delivers up to *you*. Ask for a picture of the way you once were and how you can be again.

See yourself erect and radiantly healthy.

Are you having a problem giving up a certain food?

A rather drastic technique of auto-suggestion is available to you. Use it only after you have tried the positive suggestions described above. If they do not get rid of your desire for coffee, cake or some other taboo-for-arthritis food, then use one of the *Revulsion Methods* as follows:

- Relax. Visualize a cup of coffee. See yourself sipping it. It tastes like sewage. It is revolting.
- Relax. Visualize cake. It looks delicious from afar. But as you step closer you can see ants and worms all over it. There goes a cockroach! It is revolting.
- Relax. See yourself eating bread. It tastes like burnt rubber. You know that every time you taste bread it will taste like burnt rubber. Later, you try a bite. Sure enough it does. It is revolting to you!

I repeat. These are *last resort methods* as they are *negative* in their operation. *However*, they will serve to break the back of the health-destroying habits. Later, as the revolting suggestion wears off, as it will within a few days, you can once again try the regular suggestions with a strong likelihood of more positive results.

## Learn all you can about healthy eating

Once you have started to eat properly, your motivation to continue *must be itself continuous.*

You need to remind yourself, every time you are faced with food to eat or food to buy, the truths about nutrition and especially the harrowing truths about processed foods.

Health foods are now in the headlines. New discoveries about what is happening to our ecological habitat called Earth are made almost daily. There is plenty to read about the pros and cons of organic and natural foods.

One story appeared about how a Honolulu natural-food restaurant was catering entire dinner parties of natural or organic foods for the hostess who wants to enjoy her own party. Their *piéce de resistance* or main course was a buffet green salad beautifully garnished with alfalfa sprouts, avocado, and a half dozen raw fresh vegetables. Guests had fun mixing their own blended juices from trays of fresh fruits and vegetables.

Hardly a day goes by when a new book is not published on the subject, like *Healing Foods Cookbook* by Jane Sen, or *Nutritional Health Bible* by Linda Lazarides.

For decades we have been bombarded with 'information' by the food processors. It is still continuing. But now at least we can get the other side of the story and put things in their proper perspective. We can remind ourselves that 'enriched' means first denatured, then partially restored; that attractive colouring in food should not be accepted as a 'come-on', but instead as a 'put-off' and that such hardsell motivators as 'quick,' 'easy,' 'smooth,' 'improved' are really red warning flags flying in the wind of blowhard writers. The worm has turned. And in the process it is aerating the earth for natural growth.

As more and more people frequent health-food stores and discover new vibrant tastes of living food, they educate their taste buds to what is good for them and they recognize empty calories and the products of depleted soils. They demand fresh products from supermarkets. They inquire if these have been sprayed.

"Do you have any organically grown vegetables?"

"What is the meaning of sodium diacetate on this package?"

This is the process of motivation through education that promises to change our world for the better.

## The warning signs of arthritis

On the other side of the educational coin is the need to know more about arthritis. What types are there? Are the approaches to cure different? Is the prognosis for permanent cure better for one kind than another?

There are advance warnings when we close to arthritis. Nature's pre-arthritis signs are blessings if we notice them, tragedies if we don't.

### Bursitis

Here are some of the warnings.

Around our major joints like the shoulders and hips there are numerous little ball-bearing-like sacs. Their function is to permit the muscles of the joint to work smoothly so that the joint can go through its full range of motion with ease.

If these little ball bearings aren't fed the nutrients they need for proper function, they let us know by becoming painful when we move in certain ways. It may be that the pain only comes on when we extend our arm fully or when we lift something. Assuming no correction in the food supply takes place, pain will now begin when the arm is raised only half-way. Since the arm cannot be raised all the way, adhesions form around the joint and it becomes impossible to put it through its full range of motion.

Now, it may become necessary to put the patient under anaesthesia and forcibly break these adhesions. If adequate diet isn't instituted at this point, and if exercise isn't maintained to prevent adhesions from re-forming, the joint again returns to only half function, or less.

The hip joint acts similarly. Only here we seldom put the hip joint through its full range of motion in normal usage as we do our arm. The hip and shoulder joints are ball joints. They should be able to swing in an arc. No one actually puts his hip joint through its full range of motion. That is why bursitis can sneak up on us. One day we find that, just in walking, the joint becomes painful.

The pain from bursitis of the hip will go down as far as the *outside* of the calf, never in the back of the calf and into the foot as in sciatica. The treatment for bursitis is entirely different from the treatment for sciatica.

Bursitis is a prearthritic condition caused by inflammation of the bursa around the hip joint. It can be caused by low back sprain, arthritis of the lumbar vertebra, or even by constipation.

Tendonitis (inflammation of a tendon) and myositis (inflammation of a muscle) are so closely allied as to be considered one disease. The cause here is the same as in bursitis. Frankly, these three should not be considered separately. It is highly improbable that any one of these conditions will be found existing independently. So, the treatment for one is the same as the treatment for all.

## Fatigue

There is a cardinal symptom that precedes arthritis. It is always present, even in cases of acute rheumatoid arthritis. It is fatigue. This is where tendonitis, bursitis, or myositis do not get a chance to warn you.

Fatigue is a common pre-existing symptom of all arthritics. Now, of course, everyone who suffers from chronic fatigue does not develop arthritis, but everyone who develops arthritis has suffered and does suffer from fatigue. Fatigue is indeed one of the earliest precursors or signs of arthritis.

## Blood changes

There are two other signs that are fairly constant before arthritis sets in. A check should be made to determine if they exist when fatigue is a constant companion.

One is a lowering of the amount of haemoglobin, or oxygen-carrying power of the blood, usually to around 70 per cent, when 100 per cent is normal.

The other is a high-blood sedimentation rate.

Normally, when blood is withdrawn from a vein and placed in a glass tube, with a solution in it, the red blood cells settle to the bottom of the tube slowly in one hour. For a normal reading, the cells should settle out to 10 on the scale. In prearthritic conditions, as well as in arthritis, the cells settle out 20 or more, even up to and over 100, an hour. One of my arthritic patients settled out at 154 in an hour.

Progress in the treatment of arthritis can be fairly well gauged by the doctor noticing a steady improvement in the sedimentation rate. That is, at the start of the treatment, if the sedimentation rate is 50, and as treatment progresses, the rate falls to 40, 30, 20, etc., definite improvement is taking place. At the same time, the percentage of haemoglobin rises, getting closer to 100 per cent each time it is taken.

Haemoglobin levels are often shown as milligrams per 100 millilitres of blood. The normal is 12-15mg/100ml falling to 9-10mg/100ml. These changes are more common in rheumatoid arthritis. In osteoarthritis the blood haemoglobin and the ESR (erythrocyte sedimentation rate) may remain normal.

## The many faces of arthritis – are they really one?

Arthritis is being produced in the laboratory. Rats, cats, and dogs are being given arthritis by controlled diets that are nutritionally deficient.

One experiment with cats was conducted by Dr Francis Pottenger of the University of California at Berkeley. He fed the cats cooked meat and cooked milk. The cats developed arthritis on this diet. They even died of it. The more the meat and milk were cooked, the quicker the cats developed arthritis.

A controlled group of cats was fed on raw milk and raw meat. These cats never developed arthritis. They were playful, happy, and healthy

This is a very important experiment in the search for the cause and cure of arthritis. But it is rejected by many researchers because they cannot see why cooking anything can be a cause of any disease. After all, they say, haven't we been cooking food for centuries? You know, or will know, differently

When your pain, heat, and swelling disappears in a few days on a diet of uncooked, unprocessed foods, you won't particularly care *why* it happened in your joy and relief that it *has* happened.

Just why this happens, or why cooked food or processed food can cause arthritis, is for experts like Dr Pottenger to determine. I suppose many doctors don't know exactly how aspirin works, yet they prescribe it! They should also prescribe the diet in this book whether or not science has yet come up with the whys and the wherefores.

*Know the warning signs of arthritis and you can head off the siege of pain that might otherwise be your lot.*

Also, know the symptoms of arthritis and you can get a head start dissolving the condition *before* it makes headway

## Confusing names for arthritis

Over the years, physicians have been confusing themselves, and the public by attaching a great many names to arthritis.

We have called *osteoarthritis* by such names as: Hyperthropic Arthritis, Degenerative Arthritis, and Marie Strümpell's Disease, to mention a few.

Likewise, *rheumatoid arthritis* has been called Chronic Infectious Arthritis, Atrophic Arthritis, Prolific Arthritis, and Arthritis Deformans.

## Different forms of arthritis

The term *arthritis* means *inflammation of the joint*. Medical experts have identified more than one hundred conditions that meet this criterion, and are therefore classified as forms of arthritis. These include lupus, gout, and ankylosing spondylitis; fortunately, these conditions are rare. Osteoarthritis and rheumatoid arthritis are the most common forms of the disease, affecting many millions of people around the world.

Both osteoarthritis and rheumatoid arthritis cause joints to become hot, painful, and to swell. The pain is fairly constant if the joint is at rest. It becomes more intense when the joint is called upon to bend, or move, and becomes extremely intense if it has to bear weight.

That is their basic similarity. Their basic difference is this: in osteoarthritis the bones seem to wear down at the joints. In rheumatoid arthritis there is inflammation and bony overgrowth.

*Osteoarthritis of the fingers* produces a typical deformity. If the disease strikes the index finger, it causes the last joint to bend toward the middle finger, and if it attacks the pinky, it causes that finger to bend toward the middle finger. It's peculiar but osteoarthritis, when attacking the fingers, never causes either the index finger or the pinky to turn away from the middle finger, always towards it.

Here's another peculiarity of osteoarthritis. When it attacks the *hip joints*, bony absorption takes place both in the ball of the thigh bone and in the cup-like process the ball fits into. Any movement of the hip becomes painful.

The *Knee joints* present a different picture. Here there seems to be a combination of both osteoarthritis and rheumatoid arthritis at work to destroy the joint. There is both an absorption and, at the same time, an increase of the bone development around the joint.

Another interesting fact about the knees is that if only one is involved, it is invariably the left! When both are involved, the left is afflicted much more frequently than the right.

All joints can become involved with rheumatoid arthritis. One thing that we can surely say is that rheumatoid arthritis does not respect any joint. It even attacks the jaw. That is one joint osteoarthritis leaves alone.

Acute rheumatoid arthritis is often called rheumatic fever. This is one of the most feared diseases of this arthritis group. At the same time, it responds most dramatically, and most rapidly, to proper treatment.

In fact, this disease can be readily brought under control in three to ten days. Heat and pain vanish. Swelling of the involved joints diminishes dramatically.

There is no excuse to have those afflicted with this disease suffer any longer. There is no excuse, if proper preventive dietary measures are instituted, for this disease to attack anyone.

In spinal arthritis, Spondylitis, or Marie Strümpell's Disease, which are all the same, there is again a destruction of the bones as well as an increase of bone production, together with – heat.

So it is very hard, in many of these cases, to name the condition either *osteoarthritis* or *rheumatoid arthritis*.

Usually, we physicians call it osteoarthritis.

## One step to change for old or young

"I'm too old to change."

"How can I stop eating toast and drinking coffee after 60 years of these breakfasts?"

"Hot oatmeal is a tradition in our family. So are Sunday pancakes."

Everybody can change his eating habits. For some it's easy, some hard. All you have to do is to start your change.

The day you make a change for good health you have started a dynamic reconditioning process. The new begins to take the place of the old.

Every day it becomes easier, more natural. Memory of old taste favourites fades away and new favourites take their place.

### The case history of a 73-year-old

Take Mr H. A. At 73 he had severe destructive arthritis of the right hip. He needed two crutches to walk. He liked his beer. Doughnuts and coffee were sometimes all he ate till dinner. Talk about habits, he just could not see himself living any differently. He had even grown used to the crutches – but not the pain. It was the pain that brought him to me.

He shook his head at the diet. He had never liked salad. He could not remember the taste of peaches raw, as the canned syrupy variety was one of his staples. But even with crutches a step was excruciating.

He found there was one good thing about the diet right away: no preparation needed. It was just about as easy as the cans and the boxes. Then the pain started to leave. He had no need of self-hypnotism, auto-suggestion, the revolting techniques, or any other habit-changing device.

The blessing of painless steps changed his deeply ingrained eating habits.

Still he had to start. Since Mr H. A. suffered arthritis only in the right hip, X-rays showed a substantial difference between the right and left joints. There was no rounded ball in the right hip. It was parallel, flat. In contrast the left hip was nearly normal. Three months later, X-rays showed that the joint is not yet recovered or rebuilt, but he could walk without crutches. And without pain.

## Why has this diet gone so long undiscovered?

The answer to the above question is it *has* been previously discovered. Many used to eat this way regularly.

Most doctors feel they have a duty to make 'civilized' ways work. They feel that to go back to 'pre-civilized' methods of health is unscientific.

Still, osteoarthritis has been found in some fossils of prehistoric man, indicating that foods necessary for the prevention of arthritis were not always available to him.

Occasionally, modem medical practitioners are courageous enough to make the dietary truths they understand known to the public.

Dr DeForest Clinton Jarvis, who revealed the folk-medicine practices of Vermont in his books *Folk Medicine* and *Arthritis and Folk Medicine*, pointed his finger at wheat foods, white sugar, pasteurized milk, muscle meats, and citrus fruits as new factors in our environment which were causing unwanted changes in the body.

In his 1968 book *There Is a Cure for Arthritis*, Paavo O. Airola, N.D., revealed the high incidence of success in a Swedish clinic where fasting was the chief therapy and processed foods never crossed the threshold. Here, too, fresh fruits, juices, and salads were the order of the day.

Scores of medical doctors are researching the files of the Association for Research and Enlightenment in Virginia Beach where the works of the famous 'Sleeping Prophet,' Edgar Cayce, are recorded. Those whose interest is arthritis find that Cayce, too, pointed the finger at white flour, carbonated drinks, alcohol, and such other stimulants as coffee and tea. He found elimination a prime factor and in his diets for arthritis it was common to find raw fruits and raw vegetables, nuts, berries, and salads. Lamb, fish, and fowl were the main sources of protein, with liver and tripe often given special mention.

Although Dan Dale Alexander, author of *Arthritis And Common Sense*, emphasized foods that lubricate the joints, he came up with a number of dietary parallels. He found against citrus fruits, against tea, and against the usual methods of drinking coffee, against carbonated drinks, against sugar. He found in favour of milk, tossed salads, cod liver oil, raw vegetables, and other factors on our list.

All of these men did what they could, just as I am doing, to cure arthritis and to make the cure known to the world.

## The rise of consumerism may lead to the downfall of arthritis

Fortunately, there is a better chance today that the dietary approach to arthritis will be accepted. The reason is the rise of 'consumerism.'

The average person used to swallow everything that he was fed. Today he knows better.

He knows that high-powered lobbyists are interfering with the best intentions of government to safeguard the food we eat.

He knows that the permissiveness toward substances or chemicals that cause no short-term ill effects has been an error. 'No short-term effects' can still mean 'fatal long-term effects.'

He knows that the environment is now partially hostile to his survival and he must be discriminating in what he eats, drinks, breathes, wears, and touches.

Who was it said "no institution has within itself the power to reform, change, or transform itself"? Certainly an age of change is upon us. The institution of government is feeling the stress and strains of change. So is the institution of education. And so is the institution of health care.

But don't leave the burden of change on them. You must be the one to change. Change must start with you. You must decide to be discriminating in what you eat.

This responsibility is yours. You are the sole master of the situation. You can continue to sit back with arthritis, feel sorry for yourself, and be the creature of circumstances. Or ...

You can be the creator of your circumstances. You can create circumstances characterized not by pain, misery, incapacitation, worry, fatigue, and despair. Rather you can create circumstances that are characterized by good health, energy, vitality, optimism, enthusiasm, and an infectious joy of living. To create these new circumstances in your life you must change your eating habits.

The bountiful rewards of health should be motivation enough. If, however, you find the mind is willing but the body resists, use self-hypnosis, educate yourself by reading the latest environmental news and discoveries, or use whatever habit-changing techniques you have found successful in the past.

I promise you one thing: Start, and you will never want to go back to your painful life again. Your happiness will be too valuable to exchange for a cup of coffee and a piece of cake.

## For your action

- Do the relaxation programme in this chapter. When you are deeply relaxed give yourself the mental image suggestions that make new eating habits effortless for you. If you have a problem with a particular food use the powerful revulsion technique to break its hold over you.
- See yourself free of pain. See the body's restorative powers bringing renewal to your bones and joints.
- Educate yourself about the environment. This will convince you of the need to be discriminating in choice of food and drink in order to survive in good health.

# CHAPTER 5

# Easy Ways to Hasten Your Cure Through Better Elimination

The old-time family doctor understood the importance of proper elimination more than it is appreciated today. It is not a pleasant subject, but this chapter will teach you to know your body better and how to help it help itself. Proper elimination, quickly and fully, can be controlled. It is as important as diet to your arthritis cure.

I'll wager that if you have arthritis your organs of elimination are sluggish.

*Part of the reason that two people can eat the same foods and only one of them get arthritis is that the other is doing a better job of eliminating the poisons.*

When the poisons are not quickly and totally ejected by the body the resulting toxic condition can bring on arthritis and a host of other ailments.

One of the reasons why you must fast on the first day of your cure is to help your organs of elimination catch up on their vital task.

But then you must do what you can to help these organs stay current in the days following the fast. That's what this chapter is all about. It concerns another important way to maintain youthfulness in the bodily functions – for healthy joints without arthritis pain.

## Why arthritis slows you down

A colleague of mine pointed to a store executive who was busy with a customer, talking to someone else on the phone, and answering a pricing problem posed by a sales person ... all at the same time. "There's a potentially sick man," he remarked. Several weeks later that man was suddenly stricken with ...

No, not arthritis. He suffered a heart attack.

Arthritis creeps up on you. It is usually below the level of pain and observable symptoms for at least a short while before it emerges as a full-blown case.

During this period, the person is anything but energetic. He would not be likely to exhibit the kind of excessive nervous energy that the store executive did.

The person about to get arthritis slows down in his body activities. Then when arthritis arrives, he slows down further. And, as you know, he can come to a complete forcible stop.

What causes the body to slow down to begin with?

As you know, there are two major roadblocks that we throw in the body's way:

- Tension
- Poor nutrition.

When we are tense about financial or personal problems, or experience chronic worry, we are taking energy away from its normal physical duties and expending it in this negative, unproductive way. We are also causing abnormal constrictions in the body that make more energy necessary – while we actually unconsciously allow it less.

*Result: The body's functions do not have the energy they need to perform at their normal, healthy rate. They slow up.*

Also, when we do not feed the body properly, either by giving it fewer of the nutrients it needs or more of the poisons it must work to eliminate, the body slows up. It is just what happens to your car when you take your foot off the accelerator. The fuel supply diminishes. The motor slows down. When you eat the wrong foods, you are cutting off fuel, and you are also adding poisons, giving your 'car' an uphill road to climb on less gas.

*Result: The body's organs do not have the nutrients they need to perform an even heavier task. They slow up.*

This slowing-up process of the body includes the muscles of the intestines. They no longer work at peak efficiency. Elimination of body wastes is slowed. As elimination is slowed, poisons can be *reabsorbed*\* by the bloodstream, further affecting the efficiency of the body's functions. It can have a snowballing effect, with things getting progressively worse. That is, unless you do something to reverse the cycle.

Suppose you have removed by surgery a 'joint mouse' – an abnormal bone growth due to osteoarthritis. It is no longer there. Yet the osteoarthritis remains. It can grow another 'joint mouse.'

Remove the poisons and putrefaction from the intestines that are the by-product of constipation. The constipation remains. It creates more poisons in its place.

So it is with colonic irrigation. It does not remove the constipation.

Still, just as the surgery may have been a helpful if temporary expedient, so enemas can serve to cleanse the body temporarily as you work on the cure. They help the body to reverse the cycle.

Soon the slowdown ends. The build-up begins.

## Nature's best laxative

"Is irregularity robbing your todays of their fullest enjoyment?" Such a laxative ad has strong appeal. Advertisers know how to 'reach' the person whose slowed-down processes of elimination make him feel sluggish and held down.

Laxatives do the job. They do it again and again. In fact, you must use them again and again to do the job. That is the trouble with laxatives.

Some laxatives depend on a stimulating effect. What they do is annoy the living daylights out of the intestinal walls to create that extra push that moves the waste material out of the body. What happens when you whip a horse to make it move? Soon it won't move unless you do whip it. The whipping does not give energy to

---

\* The accumulation of poisons in the blood and tissues occurs more as a result of the reduced rate of absorption into the intestines owing to slow elimination than to reabsorption from the intestines. The effect is still the same.

the horse. It just looks that way. In fact, the whipping may be weakening the horse.

## Artificial laxatives' dangers

The laxatives that provide this kind of stimulating effect perpetuate their own need. After prolonged use the body does not function well without them even after the cause of the constipation has long since passed.

Other laxatives work by their own special physical qualities. Some swell up in the intestines. Others absorb moisture, releasing it in the lower intestines. Some lubricate.

They all work because they pose some kind of problem to the body. I don't recommend them as a way of life because we are throwing enough unnatural conditions at the body as it is. You may take a laxative at this early stage in the treatment temporarily, if you insist. I recommend one half ounce of phosphate of soda in water as the least harmful of the artificial laxatives.

Some laxatives, like mineral oil, will prevent the absorption of nutrients and vitamins by the oil-coated membranes of the intestines. Some provide an added load on the liver or other digestive organs. They are largely weakening rather than strengthening.

## Nature's laxatives are best

What then can a person do?

Remember the theme of *Blue Bird* by Maeterlinck? The story characters searched far and wide for the treasure, then found it in their own back yard. They weren't looking for a laxative. But we are. And that is exactly where we find nature's perfect laxative. In our own 'back yard.'

Raw vegetables and fruits are nature's answer. And in its infinite wisdom, *nature has provided with its proper food exactly what the body needs for its proper elimination.*

So, you see, the seven-day programme to rid your joints of heat, swelling, and pain will also encourage your body to restore its own natural regularity. First, there's the fast that allows rest and a catching-up period. Then come all those crisp, juicy, raw fruits and vegetables.

You can't miss with this natural laxative system.

Let me repeat the instructions for the charcoal and corn test here in more detail. It is vital to your cure that your bowels are currently and normally active.

### The charcoal test

At the end of an evening meal take six charcoal tablets. You can obtain these from your local chemist. Take them with water or unsweetened prune or grape juice. These tablets can be swallowed whole, without chewing, or pulverized and the powder taken with a little liquid.

The charcoal tablets will colour your stool black. The entire black should be eliminated the following morning, from 12 to 14 hours after its ingestion. This might surprise you, but sometimes it takes arthritics four days to a week before it shows and is completely eliminated. Don't ever wait that long. Take an enema promptly and get rid of the charcoal.

### The corn test

The next night you can check again by taking one or two ears of corn with your evening meal, purposely not chewing all kernels. If you cannot get fresh corn on the cob, cook frozen raw corn. The undigested kernels should, as with the charcoal, be completely eliminated the following morning, or within 12 to 14 hours.

Once again, if the corn does not show as it should, the same procedure with the enemas, or colonic irrigation, should be undertaken to get all the kernels out as you did with the charcoal.

### The beetroot test

By the second day, you will have learned whether or not you are constipated. A third material you can add to this sequence is beetroot. Cook two small beetroots with the skin on in a small amount of water, and eat them with the skin still on. The next day you should see the characteristic blood-red colour and the skin should be seen in your stool. In the vast majority of arthritis cases, constipation is present.

## Recommendations for constipation

If you are constipated, here is what I recommend:

- Take a safe laxative from your health-food store. The bulk-action type, which train the muscles of your colon, are best. Do not use any laxative steadily – change frequently.
- Eat bulk fruits (raw).

Avoid harsh laxatives as they may cause problems. Ask your chemist or doctor to recommend one that suits your needs. Lactulose is often recommended for its gentleness, but even this has the drawback of causing wind and cramps in some people.

### Bulk fruits

What are bulk fruits? These include dried or fresh prunes or figs, unsulphured, of course, and with no other preservatives added (such as sodium or calcium propionate). These also include apples and pears, which are around most of the year, and the more seasonal peaches, nectarines, and plums, as well as such berries in season as blueberries, blackberries, and mulberries.

When sluggish bowel action is delayed three or more days, take a dish of prunes daily, or six to 12 figs daily, or two apples daily. Take the phosphate of soda, also.

As bowel action approaches four times a day or when the charcoal or corn kernels begin to show up within 12 to 14 hours, reduce the laxative and rely more and more on the bulk fruits.

There is no harm in making this charcoal and corn test every few days until the process of elimination proves to be current. Nor is there any harm in checking yourself from time to time when you are free of your pain and feeling your young self again. Just remember to alternate between charcoal the first night and corn the next. Then take an enema after waiting to see what the time factor measures.

## Aids for chronic constipation

Some people have been constipated for 30 years or more. They will require constant vigilance for several months in overcoming their condition. The reason is that their large bowel or colon becomes distended.

Normally, this large bowel or colon is about two inches in diameter and about six feet long. If it is not emptied regularly, every 24 hours at least, then the next-day's waste is shoved into it. Sometimes it has to accommodate two, three, or four days' waste.

Storing instead of eliminating causes the colon to stretch in diameter and in length.

I have seen the colon extended over four inches in diameter and nine feet in length, able to hold waste for a week. Can you imagine what these people's health experiences were? You can never cure your arthritis while this condition of aggravated constipation is permitted to continue.

As I said before, it can take months in such cases for the bowel muscles to shrink down closer to normal size. But you must persevere. Anything short of complete elimination of one day's waste by the following morning just will not make the grade for arthritis cure. Allowing the waste from one breakfast to remain in the body for 24 hours or more just won't do.

Some foods will colour your stool and eliminate the need for a charcoal or corn test. Examples are spinach and red beets. If you have a meal with spinach on Monday evening the dark green should show up in the stool by Tuesday evening.

Is this a new concept to you? I'll wager it is. Most of us go through life stuffing food in one end and not knowing or caring how long it takes to emerge from the other end. Yet it is vitally important that people with arthritis become aware of these two ends of the alimentary tract.

Your programme is:

- Test.
- Take a laxative.
- Eat raw bulk fruits.

- Keep testing.
- And help nature with an internal bath.

## Both good nutrition and good elimination are needed to cure arthritis

A woman came back from an expensive health spa still suffering from arthritis and when I gave her the details of the diet cure she rose up on her haunches and protested, "But, doctor, I was just on a diet like that and it didn't work." When she told me about the spa, I asked her if they gave her colonic irrigations. "Oh, it wasn't that kind of place."

You must transform your home into that kind of a place. The bathroom is as important as the kitchen.

## A case history of 24-year-old H.M.

H.M. came to me when he was 24. But let's let him tell his own story:

"My fight against arthritis started when I was 17. I first felt less free motion of my spine that gradually aggravated. On and off I had inflammation in my spine. Finally, when I was 23, I began to notice some deformity. The lower back pain came more often. All these years I had been seeing orthopaedists who couldn't help me a bit.

"Then I learned about Dr Campbell. After three days my inflammation at the spine was gone completely. With the help of an intake of nutritious food like seafood, fruit, bone marrow, and vegetables, and taking care of my bowel every day, I can now establish motion in most of my joints in the spine.

"Dr Campbell's way to control arthritis is the most convincing one for me, and I wish everybody who suffers from this dreadful disease could know this way to far better health."

I think the important words in this statement are, "taking care of my bowel every day." People are loath to talk about this subject, much less do something about it. The arthritis cure is more likely to be called a diet cure than an elimination cure.

Of course, it is both.

It is useless to go on the diet and not take the necessary steps to correct sluggish elimination.

It is just as useless to correct the elimination but not the diet.

When you do both, that body of yours is going to feel like new.

## The internal bath – helping nature

In time, raw fruits and raw vegetables will cleanse your innards of the putrefaction brought about by unnatural foods and the imbalance they bring to your body.

There are ways to help nature along and to decrease that time period. One way is the internal bath we talked about earlier – otherwise known as the enema.

I'm not about to convince you that enemas can be fun. Far from it. But they need not be the awkward, uncomfortable act that we remember them to be. I am going to give you a procedure that will make your colonic irrigation easier, more natural, and more routine. But don't let it become a regular routine because here, too, the body can develop a dependency.

You owe it to yourself to help nature to help you in the beginning. After all, consider who it has been that interfered in the first place. Then you also owe it to yourself to let your body take over the natural way.

Even if the charcoal and corn test shows you are eliminating in less than 15 hours, one or two enemas can be helpful in ridding the intestinal walls of stubborn putrefied material that may be clinging.

There is no point in covering all the wrong ways to take an enema. One will suffice. The most frequent mistake is to sit on the commode, insert the nozzle in the rectum and let the water run in. This, frankly, is a real douche, not an enema.

### How to take an enema

To take an enema properly, fill a two-quart bag or can with warm water. Test it by placing your finger in it. It should not feel cool or hot, just warm to the finger.

*Procedure*: Hang up the enema bag about two to three feet above you. Lie down on the floor or bed, on your left side, with the right knee over the left. The left arm should rest along the left side. With the right hand grasping it, hold the hose near its well-lubricated nozzle. Control the flow by pinching the rubber tube. You can do this by intertwinning it around the right index finger and squeezing the thumb and middle finger against the index finger. This will permit you to control the volume of water that enters the rectum. You can pause, continue the flow, pause.

Keep the flow going in this manner until you feel the first urge to eliminate. Stop the flow and get up and expel what you can. When you feel that you have completely expelled the contents, lie down again and repeat. In fact, you should refill the bag with water of the same temperature and repeat the performance.

Continue to refill the bag, and run the water in, until you come to the point where the evacuation consists only of discoloured water.

### Enemas should be only temporarily used

Fortunately, enemas and extremely restricted diets are not part of your future life style. You should be free of the need to subject yourself to both in a very short time compared to the permanency of crippling, painful arthritis.

Meanwhile, I am going to help you help your other organs of elimination to normalize. Don't worry – no awkward, unappetizing procedures.

### Warning about enemas

Today, enemas are used primarily as an aid to medical treatment or diagnosis. Few experts share Dr Campbell's enthusiasm for the use of self-administered enemas (colonic irrigation) to clean the bowel. Such procedures may create an imbalance in the body's normal chemical balance, and could damage delicate tissues. You can successfully use this diet without subjecting yourself to this procedure.

## Your other organs of elimination

Show me a person suffering with arthritis and I'll show you a person suffering from constipation, whose breath is anything but fresh, whose skin is sandy dry and whose urine is dark amber in colour and doubly odorous.

When these people improve their bowel movement, they improve all of these other symptoms, too. Because these are all signs of an overloaded elimination system, – signs of overloaded lungs, skin, and kidneys.

When the bowels do not function as they should, the liquid waste from the delayed, decaying faecal material is reabsorbed. This means it is picked up by the blood stream and carried to the kidneys, skin, and lungs.

### The kidneys

When the sluggish bowels place a continuous overload on the kidneys, the urine shows it. It becomes concentrated and turns darker in colour.

The kidneys begin to work overtime. There is an increased frequency of urination. Often this is noticed when coffee, beer, or liquor is consumed. These are toxic materials to the body and the role of disposing them is assigned normally to the kidneys. We are told to call these liquids diuretics or kidney stimulants. What a travesty!

When the kidneys are subjected to this type of overload over an extended time, a lowered resistence to bacterial infection can take place. To help prevent this a gram of natural vitamin C (bioflavonoid complex) should be taken daily. Parsley tea or unsweetened barley water also cleanses the kidneys and bladder.

Meanwhile, the skin is showing the strain, too.

As the kidneys fall behind on the job that needs to be done, the skin is utilized by the body to help out. The result is that perspiration becomes offensive. No amount of deodorant can alleviate the odour for more than a few minutes.

## The skin

This can be just a passing phase. The skin is a willing helper to the bowels and the kidneys, but not too well equipped to do the job. Soon the skin 'cops out.' It no longer operates properly as an organ of elimination. It becomes dry and sandy to the touch as the sweat and sebaceous glands act like a 'stuck team' – those horses who have been whipped too hard, once too often, and now refuse to work at all.

In acute rheumatoid arthritis the skin is extremely dry with a sandy feeling. There is generally no apparent moisture except in the palms of the hands and soles of the feet. The rest of the skin areas have that coarse feeling.

To aid the eliminative function of the skin, hot tub baths, which increase perspiration, are in order. These should be administered daily or even twice daily, if it does not weaken the patient. If steam baths are available locally, these, too, help to open pores and induce perspiration.

Here is another very important point for those who have Marie Strümpell's disease, or spondylitis. If the disease is caught early enough, say within the first five years, it can be brought under control rapidly by this treatment system and no further ankylosis (destruction of a joint by overgrowth of bone) takes place.

The body odour in victims of this disease is invariably very offensive and the skin, especially over the spine, emits a clammy, sticky sweat.

The spine itself is hot. The skin over that area of the back involved has a noticeable increase in warmth while the skin of the entire back has that peculiar clammy feel. This abnormal perspiration changes to normal as the disease is brought under control.

In these cases, it is advisable for the patient to take one tablespoon of powdered brewers' yeast and one tablespoon of black strap molasses three times a day until the body sweat becomes normal or there is no longer any offensive odour. A couple of ounces of heavy cows' cream can be added to the above mixture for good taste and good measure.

### The lungs

Lungs are important organs of elimination. Their primary function is to get rid of carbon dioxide and at the same time supply oxygen for all the billions of cells in the body.

Deep breathing permits oxygen to be carried into the lowest recesses of the lungs, thus exposing as many red blood cells as possible to oxygen. Once the oxygen is absorbed, the haemoglobin of the red blood cells transfers this life-giving oxygen to the cells for their survival and repair

Most of us do not take a deep breath from one week to the next, unless we are put under physical stress. As you can guess, anybody with rheumatoid arthritis had better take a few Deep breathing exercises are of definite value to help the overall purification process.

In addition to carrying oxygen to the red blood cells and getting rid of carbon dioxide, there are other waste gases thrown off by the lungs. In arthritis there is an extra burden placed on the lungs as on all organs of elimination.

You can help your lungs. Do deep breathing and exercise physically, to your tolerance, to help increase the flow of blood to the lungs, as well as to the rest of the body.

Deep breathing should be done outdoors if possible or with the windows open. The object is to fill your lungs with the purest air and that richest in oxygen. Pure air is a rare commodity these days. If you face a heavily used thoroughfare go to the back of the house where fumes are not likely to be as bad.

Try to make this an hourly habit. Take six to ten deep breaths, filling your lungs with oxygen, then breathing out to expel as much air as you can.

There is no need to rush this. Pause. Take your time and enjoy it.

---

**A case history of relief**

"It must be something like a virus that's bugging me," said the 35-year-old woman who worked as a clerk in a bank. "My joints ache and I have an unmistakable body odour."

It was no virus. I told her so. I asked her to go on the arthritis diet. She was indignant.

"Doctor, I'm young. This can't be arthritis. It's some kind of a bug."

She refused to go on the diet. I don't know what happened over the next three months but I can imagine the miracle drugs she must have consumed in search of the villainous virus. When she came to my office again, the arthritis was painfully obvious. She couldn't count money out and had to take a leave of absence from her job.

"I think it is arthritis," she admitted. "But how could it happen to me?"

I asked her what she had been eating typically. Then I explained how it could happen to her. She then attended to her elimination. She went on the diet of fresh fruit and fresh vegetables. She was back riffling money in two weeks.

Some do not have it so easy. Millions of people have sat in a doctor's office as he looked over X-rays and shaking his head, said, "Your arthritis is obviously getting worse. I presume the pain is no better." Then the discussion turns to rest, mild exercise, the possibility of surgery in the future.

Year after year.

It's no fun taking enemas, checking your stool, giving up foods that you have been used to eating.

But arthritis is no fun either, especially when it becomes a life style.

## For your action

- Take a laxative to help clear out accumulated poisons at the outset. Alternate the laxatives from time to time. Do not depend on any one continuously. Ultimately you must rely upon the raw bulk fruits and raw vegetables.
- Test yourself repeatedly with the charcoal and corn, flushing with enemas when the period is noted. If all waste is not

eliminated from the day before, give yourself these enemas until this period of elimination is reached.

- Help your kidneys with the parsley tea if they need it, your skin with the hot baths if it needs a perspiration assist, and your lungs with the deep breathing.
- Be aware of elimination as a prerequisite to a purified, arthritis-free body.

# CHAPTER 6

# Ten Fun Minutes a Day to Regain
# Lost Movements of Your Body

Moving the body in certain ways can help speed your recovery. Let's not call these 'exercises' because they are really quite different. You can enjoy some of these motions in bed or in an overstuffed chair. They are never tiring and some do not even require expenditure of your own energy

Some foods contain powerful medicines which may be aggravating your arthritis. Chicken or beef may have had medicines injected in the creature for faster growth and for greater resistance to microbes ready to invade their bodies weakened by processed food.

You think you are enjoying finger-licking good chicken or tender roast beef. What you are really enjoying may be an indirect dose of stilboestrol, arsenic, or aureomycin.

Your body does not easily recover from these. Even when the heat, pain, and swelling leave, thanks to the fresh raw fruits and vegetables and the organ meats, all is not over. A delicate chemical balance remains in your body The pain may have left you ten days ago. But it can return in ten hours!

Every day that you treat your body with the proper unprocessed, natural, nutritious foods you reinforce your good health and consolidate your gains.

Yet I have seen a man 'reward' himself for a week of faithful adherence to proper diet by taking a small piece of chocolate. Within 24 hours he had a recurrence of that familiar but dreaded stiffness in his fingers and legs.

Reward indeed!

This chemical balance is that delicate because we have, in effect, used up nature's usually generous factor of safety by our continuous abuse of our body. Nature responds favourably to our return to proper foods and nutrients, but not with her usual generosity. She places us on probation.

Of course every case differs depending on the foods previously consumed, the body's tolerance for toxins, and other individual variables. But play it safe, for your own good. You can be a sure winner if you stick to the rules of healing nutrition.

Stay off the forbidden foods without exception. Stay on the original diet as long as you can, even after the pain, swelling, and heat are gone, if you want to consolidate your gains and master your cure.

This chapter gives you more ways to consolidate gains and hasten your cure. Most of these can be done right in your own home

And they are fun to do.

## Kiss that aspirin goodbye

For most arthritics, aspirin has become a friend. It has staved off pain, brought much-needed relief.

But you have paid a high price for a poor bargain in health.

In a report published some years ago, a prominent professor of surgery was quoted as saying that aspirin kills some one thousand people a year.

### Dangers of aspirin

Experimenting on rats, this professor and his colleagues found that aspirin removes the stomach's natural protective coating of mucous secretions. This leaves the stomach lining vulnerable to the acid in the aspirin which can then penetrate the stomach walls.*

---

* Pain medications containing ibuprofen can also damage the stomach lining, and should not be substituted for aspirin.

The result very often is internal bleeding. It has been estimated that one out of every eight patients admitted to a hospital for internal bleeding is there because of aspirin. Aspirin should be banned from over-the-counter sales and be available only by prescription.

If you stick to your initial diet, you will no longer need aspirin for the pain of arthritis. But I am bringing this subject up now because you should know about these side effects of aspirin. Aspirin has become a general mode of relief for practically any pain. With the first headache or other ache that comes along, it will be natural for you to think of reaching for that friendly aspirin bottle.

Know that aspirin does not only cost money. It costs in body troubles. And that kind of trouble costs more than money. Also, it spells a possible breach in the delicate chemical balance that your healing body now has.

Your body needs to absorb all the rich nutrients it can. Pitted stomach walls and even gastric ulcers, both possible effects of aspirin, are not conducive to better absorption of the nourishment your body craves ... and must have for health.

Aspirin works against you. By '*you*' I mean the whole person.

You can find evidence that it works for part of you. It is certainly effective with pain. Some evidence is turning up that it is even more basically effective in osteoarthritis.

Let's switch the scene to Connecticut. Here some university professors have discovered an enzyme which they believe is responsible for part of the joint cartilage breakdown. It does this by viscosity or slowing up the flow of vital fluids within the cartilage. When they treat this enzyme with sodium salicylate, similar to an aspirin ingredient, this enzymatic process is retarded. They feel they have found the explanation for the reduced inflammation that often takes place when large doses of aspirin are consumed by a person with arthritis. Enzymes are able to attack the joint cartilage because it is weakened by nutritional deficiency, not by aspirin deficiency.

### The necessity for curing the whole you

I vote for large doses of raw fresh fruits and raw fresh vegetables instead of drugs, even 'harmless' ones like aspirin. It helps the whole 'you,' not just your joints at the expense of your stomach and your nutrition. I hope you will vote the same way for your general health.

We need to consolidate our health gains through correct nutrition. We need to take that delicate chemical balance of our body and increase its margin of safety.

We need to nourish our tissues and organs so that the delicate chemical balance becomes an established and healthy chemical balance.

Side effects are a common characteristic of most drugs. Ask any doctor or nurse. We cannot blame aspirin alone. Often these side effects are unimportant compared to the cure or relief obtained. So we risk them in our haste 'to feel better' somehow.

They are now finding that chloroquine or Avlochor, a drug used to treat both arthritis and malaria, can cause diseased retina of the eye. Again, it's a case of no noticeable side effects over a brief period. But those who take the drug for months are risking changes in the retina and optic nerve which can produce night blindness, loss of vision in the central portion of the visual field, or even total blindness. Also, effects have been known to continue for years after the drug has been discontinued.

Are you willing to take this kind of risk?

Wouldn't you prefer a different kind of medicine where the side effects are *bonuses* instead of *penalties* and the main effect is not only relief, but *cure*?

That medicine is nature's garden and orchard bounty.

## How to circulate needed nourishment throughout your body

I have discussed one way we interfere with nature's cure. Undoubtedly, we interfere in many ways – through negative attitudes, tension, anxiety, worry. But let's get on the positive beam as follows.

There are a number of things you can do to accelerate nature's cure. I am referring now to matters beyond the intake and output – diet and elimination – discussed in previous chapters. I am now referring largely to *body motion*.

One important result of body motion is increased circulation of the blood. This helps nature because the blood is the vehicle that delivers nourishment to the body's cells, including the unhealthy cells that are causing our arthritis.

That very arthritis condition has been inhibiting your body motion, thus perpetuating its own malnutrition, aggravating your arthritis! Areas affected by arthritis can often become progressively worse due to poor blood circulation. Doctors generally recognize that mild exercise stimulates increased circulation to the weakened muscles. That it certainly does. But one step is overlooked. To the starving cell the increased blood flow is like a postman with a heavy pack, but no letter for you.

The blood is our very stream of life. It must flow normally It must bear food the body continually needs to build healthy tissue.

On its way *to* the cells, organs, and tissues of the body, the blood provides oxygen and nutrients.

On its way *from* the cells, organs, and tissues of the body, the blood carries the waste products and debris.

### Benefits of improved circulation

When we do something to help the circulation of the blood, we help our bodies two ways:

- We provide a more efficient distribution of cell nutrition.
- We provide a more efficient disposal of cell waste.

There's more to it – better disposal of cell waste means more oxygen in the cells with greater youth and vitality. But let's keep it simple ...

Let's just circulate that blood more efficiently.

Persons with arthritis are forced to be sedentary. Movement is often accompanied by pain. So arthritis sufferers lie still and sit a great deal of the time to avoid pains of movement.

### Effect of circulation on kidneys

Let's just look at the effect of this on the kidneys. Bending and twisting forces blood into 'end-of-the-line' circulation points.

Without this kind of movement, stagnant spots may develop where the smaller blood capillaries are not getting a meaningful flow of that all-important blood supply.

This is especially important in the kidneys. If the kidneys are not treated to an abundant flow of blood, they can slow down and become sluggish. Then they do not do an adequate job of getting rid of the poisonous urea which is their function.

So one thing leads to another. The extra toxins in processed food give the kidney a bigger job to do. The excess of toxins slows us down with pain, causing us to move around less. The lack of motion deprives the kidneys of the circulation they need to do even a normal job.

Result: Extra load on the kidneys leads to diminished capacity of the kidneys. We can't let this happen. We need to reverse this cycle.

Body motion is the answer. This motion helps nature circulate nourishment throughout our body. Motion helps nature flush waste and poison from everywhere in our body

## Healing body motions that we cannot call 'exercise'

'Exercise 'is a 'dirty word.' It turns people off. It conjures up an image of arms moving forward, up, forward, down, and of hands on hips, – begin!

Sitting-up exercises that are still used in many physical education programmes are exercises in futility to many people because they are so mechanical, forced, and regimented.

I'm going to try not to use the word 'exercise' because I don't wish you to engage in that kind of activity anyhow. I want you to move with a purpose – to move in ways that make you feel good. Movement and motion will be our key words in helping cure arthritis.

First, let me make it abundantly clear that even simple motions that I will now describe are not for you if your joints are still plagued with heat, swelling, and pain. Hold off these until these symptoms leave thanks to your special arthritis-curing diet and your newly efficient process of elimination.

## Specific body motions for arthritics

Here is a motion that you can enjoy while lying in bed.

Lie on your back. Raise your knees to a position that is comfortable. Now roll slightly from side to side. Use your legs to create the motion, so that the hips are involved. Don't force yourself. If there is stiffness or pain, don't go that far; even a very slight roll back and forth will be of therapeutic benefit.

Can you feel a good sensation in the lower region of your back? That's because your kidneys are getting a ten-dollar massage. You can just hear them cooing, "more, more."

*Motions, to be effective, do not have to be violent or exaggerated.* Slight motion massages those tiny capillaries and stimulates circulation just as surely as do large, energy-consuming exercises. Later you may want to engage in energetic activities, too, – the kind that make the heart pump a little harder and the respiration deepen and accelerate. But now the passive type of movements are right for you.

### The resonator factor from India

The spiritual men of India have chanted a mystical syllable for years beyond memory. It is called *Om* but vocalized like a hum: 'O-m-m-m.' It is said to be the closest that the human voice can come to imitating all the sounds in the Universe if they were heard at one time. It is used by these men to attune their bodies and minds to the forces of the Universe.

I mention it because everything in your body seems to resonate when you make this sound. Some people reportedly can make windows rattle with this sound. More important, it vibrates your whole body. You can see what I mean if you hold your hands in front of you, palms down. As you intone the sound 'O-m-m-m' you will 'hear' it with the skin of your palms. Do it again and this time feel with your fingertips the top of your head or other parts of your body. You should feel the resonating vibration. Actually you are giving yourself an internal sonic massage that is pleasant with its healing effect.

WARNING: To the person suffering from arthritis, every vibration can be painful, so here again, do not rush matters. Wait until the purification process that comes with proper diet and elimination has had time to bring you that desired relief.

## Miscellaneous circulation methods

In bed or seated in a chair, there are many movements that help your circulation. Even rocking back and forth can be good for you.

Nature has a way of inducing us to help her. When something is in our nose, we involuntarily sneeze. When something is on our skin, it is impossible to keep from scratching. Similarly, we may find ourselves unconsciously making certain movements without hands, legs, fingers, or body This is often nature's doing but it's something the body needs.

Maybe you have inhibited yourself from making such motions because they seemed silly or others might laugh. Do them now. Let yourself go. Any motion is good and if you have the idea or urge to move about in a certain way, why say "no" to your body? Say "yes." Move ... that's the important thing to do.

## Helpful motion where you need it

### Wrists

Has the heat left your wrists? If you have had arthritis of the wrists and the pain has sufficiently receded to move them around, then help nature to help you with this motion:

Let your arms hang loosely at the side of your body as you stand or as you sit in a straight-back chair. Now shake your wrists. The easiest way is to rotate the forearms quickly back and forth. Try other side-to-side or back-and-forth shaking motions, too.

This is worth doing for two or three minutes every hour. If you are in bed, do it with one wrist at a time as you let that arm dangle loosely over the side of the bed.

### Knees

If your knees have been involved in the arthritis, and the heat and pain have now receded, you can help your knees with this motion:

Sit on a table or other object high enough to permit your feet to hang loosely without touching the floor. Stretch one leg forward. Then let go and let it swing back and forth like a pendulum until it comes to rest. Try not to control the motion. Let it happen. Now do the same with the other leg. Keep doing this for two minutes every hour, increasing to three minutes as improvement is noticed.

Note that both of these activities have every right to be called motions rather than exercises. They are both done in a relaxed position, hanging limply so that muscles are not critically involved. Instead, the desired end result is movement in the joint area without muscular interference. Free motion stimulates natural circulation where it is needed most.

### Hips

Osteoarthritis of the hips calls for this type of motion – again, only after the heat leaves:

Lie on your back in bed, pointing toes upward. It takes effort to keep them pointing up, although very slight. Relax this effort. Let them fall to a natural position which is outward. Bring them back to a vertical position and let them fall outward again. Keep doing this for two or three minutes, perfecting your ability to let go and have them fall outward without any help from you.

### Spine

Those with spinal arthritis should enjoy this special motion. It is designed to flex and extend the spine gently.

While lying on the bed on your back, raise your knees against your chest as far as you can without producing pain. Fold your arms across your knees and rock your knees back and forth by the power of your arms pulling on them. Relax, pull, relax, … you'll enjoy this beneficial routine.

Continue this for two to three minutes. As time goes by gradually increase it so that you are doing it steadily for ten minutes. Enjoy this rocking motion every night and every morning.

Below is another motion worth experiencing. It extends the spine and is beneficial for everyone to stimulate the circulation.

Sit in an overstuffed chair with your knees over one arm and your back against the other arm. Now let your back bend so that it is leaning over the arm of the chair as far as it can go. The hands should dangle down behind the head with the elbows fairly straight against the ears. At the start stay in this position for 30 seconds. Straighten up, and then repeat. Keep this up, gradually extending the time you allow your back to be extended over the arm of the chair, in a relaxed position, until you can stay for three minutes without discomfort.

These are motions you should begin to enjoy a number of times a day. If possible, take a few minutes 'motion break' every hour on the hour.

You will feel, love, and live the difference.

## Movement and nutrition – the winning formula

No physical activity in the world is going to correct vitamin and mineral deficiencies or other types of nutritional shortage.

No physical activity man can devise is going to correct by itself toxic conditions caused by food additives and chemical processing.

You must not think that anything in this chapter is a substitute for raw fruits, raw vegetables, and organ meats, or that it can take the place of properly functioning organs of elimination.

### Special note

*In fact*, these physical activities can conceivably worsen the arthritis if the rules given in this book for diet and elimination are not followed. The impurities, if still there, are circulated even faster to the areas where they are being dumped by the overburdened body.

Wait until you have made some progress, evidenced by the disappearance of those arthritic heat, swelling, and pain symptoms. That is the green light for the motion routines. The blood is now freed of excess toxins and replenished with vital nutrients. It is ready to do the job right for you. Motion then helps it do that job.

First, the motions should be mild and of short duration. Later, they can be extended in both vigour and time. Still later, they can be supplemented with more general body motions that involve increased activity and muscle use. How about that? Not a mention of the word *exercise*!

## Other activities that help arthritic joints

### Walking

Walking is nature's perfect movement. It brings our entire body into the therapeutic action. At first, the walk should be a stroll. Amble along enjoying the passing scene. Rejoice in your new-found pain-free navigation.

Then use walking as a means to and a measure of your continued progress. I would like you to keep a record of your walking. Make a record of the time and approximate distance that you walk each day, always keeping your walks well below the point of fatigue. This log of your walking will reflect your improvement progress.

The log is important for you. Improvement is something that always seems to take too long. One tends to get discouraged at the slow day-to-day pace. But when you take a look at your log and see that you improved from 100 yards in ten minutes to 400 yards in 20 minutes in three-weeks time, you are indeed encouraged.

This optimistic and positive attitude of encouragement is important. Positive attitudes encourage healthy cell growth. Negative attitudes can add to health problems.

### How to check your progress

Check your progress every week. On the last day of the week you can clock the time it takes to walk the same distance you walked the first day of the week. Then go on to the longer distance you are now walking.

My problem is holding back my patients as they recover. They want to pick up all the activities they enjoyed before the onset of the arthritis, like bicycle riding, wood chopping, horse riding, and swimming.

I endorse these activities 100 per cent. But I caution against letting enthusiasm get the better of moderation. This is not always easy.

When activity is excessive in these early days or weeks of relief and progressive cure, you go beyond the desirable stimulation of circulation and provide aggravated wear and tear on newly rejuvenating joints.

Arthritic joints need more time for cure than any other part of the body. Bone growth is much slower than skin, muscle, or other tissue growth.

Have patience! Continue to move more and more, but never beyond the point of fatigue. Then, when you are your young self again, you may want to exert yourself.

## Swimming

I recommend swimming especially. After the heat leaves the joints, start swimming a few minutes a day if it is swimming weather or if there is a swimming pool available. If you do not swim, it pays to learn under competent supervision. Even if you do know how to swim, it has probably been a while since you were last swimming so that supervision might be wise at least for the first few times.

Swimming has a relaxing effect on the entire nervous system. Water massages all your body at once, giving motion to your tissues. And the cool water stimulates your circulation. It's a three-way boon to your arthritic body.

## Benefits of increased respiration

As soon as you are well enough, don't be afraid of extending yourself to increase your respiration rate. Mild jogging or other energy-consuming motion that makes you breathe just a little harder also makes the heart pump a little faster.

When the heart is 'idling,' as it is most of our sedentary life, the blood may get to all parts of the body but not in an adequate volume to do its job efficiently. Dead material or waste from living cells accumulates. If the circulation is not fast enough or in sufficient volume, it does not pick up this debris.

You will note this in 'charley horses' (a muscular binding), black and blue spots, and tender areas of the body. Pressure of accumulated debris in these spots prevents oxygen and other nutrients from getting to oxygen-starved cells.

When the heart pumps faster, it pumps with more power and produces more volume. As this 'tidal wave' of blood courses through the arteries and veins, it flushes this debris and cleanses the body internally.

So now you see the way my arthritis cure works:

- You halt the intake of chemicals and poisons.
- You nourish the body with natural, nutritious food.
- You restore normal elimination.
- You stimulate circulation with slow motion, faster motion, and finally strenuous motion.

## Motion without moving

When you expend your own energy in moving such motion is free. If, however, you would like the benefit of motion without expending your own energy you can use some electric devices. Such motion is not free; you must be ready to pay for special equipment.

### Vibratory massagers

There are various lightweight vibratory massage machines on the market. They consist of a power-driven plate which vibrates at one or two speeds. There may be extra attachments, such as rubber bulb for specific muscle areas, or spiked rubber plates for general skin stimulation.

If you, or a friend, can handle such a machine, the fine vibrations will stimulate the flow of blood when applied to muscles and ligaments around the joints. Use the plate for larger areas of stiff muscles. A word of caution: do not use a vibrator on swollen or inflamed tissues around an arthritic joint, or over varicose veins. Wait for the acute pain to disperse and use the gentle pressure movements to circulate the blood.

### Vibratory cushions

Cushions which heat up and vibrate can help the stiff back with osteoarthritis of the spine. The cushion is placed in an armchair and can be switched on for a time while you lean against it to read or watch TV.

These devices stimulate the surface blood flow and activate the deeper tissues but they are no substitute for a pair of skilled hands.

## How healing is hastened by manipulation

Suppose you were a research scientist trying to track down the cause of arthritis. Let's say you were part of the team at the Queensland Medical Research Institute in Brisbane, Australia, working on the theory that mosquitoes spread not only malaria and dengue fever but also polyarthritis. Polyarthritis causes symptoms similar to rheumatic fever or rheumatoid arthritis in its early stages. You suspect the mosquitoes of playing a part in this disease. A virus has been found in the area of an epidemic of this disease. Now you are injecting this virus into mosquitoes, allowing the virus to incubate in the mosquito a week or two and then arranging for the mosquitoes to bite mice to see if the disease can be so induced.

Now suppose somebody called to your attention that arthritis was being cured by a doctor in the United States through the use of diet. How would you feel? Would you interrupt your work? Would you feel you were wasting your time?

Chances are you would keep right on doing what you were doing. You might feel that the diet had merit, but that it was only creating a high resistance to your virus, while you would eventually find a substance to combat the virus.

So it is that some types of curative methods are bypassed or ignored in search of more germ- or virus-orientated approaches. And people go on suffering while the search continues.

One curative method that is bypassed or ignored by orthodox medicine, as well as by some manipulating osteopaths, is Osteopathic neuromuscular manipulation. This is corrective movements applied to your body by the osteopathic physician, many of whom are formally trained in these skills. The osteopath's sense of touch, if so trained, is highly sensitive. He can detect abnormal tissue long before the patient has any symptoms, or knows that trouble is coming. His hands can manipulate this abnormal tissue to increase arterial supply and venous drainage, without any painful cracking of the joints.

## Osteopathic neuromuscular manipulation

What is proper osteopathic manipulation for joints consumed with rheumatoid arthritis?

Neuromuscular manipulation is carried on above and below the relaxed joint when it is hot or acutely inflamed. This increases the blood flow to and from the joint. Repair is hastened. Pain is reduced. Motion is facilitated. And joint recovery is made possible.

The manipulating osteopath will look for complete relaxation of the joint by the patient as a prerequisite to this manipulative treatment. Part or semi-relaxation will produce only part recovery. The patient must voluntarily cooperate in producing this total relaxation.

Most small towns now enjoy the services of an osteopath. Big cities have as many as a hundred or more. If you live in a rural area, chances are there is an osteopath within a few minutes' to an hour's drive from you. Your local classified telephone directory will undoubtedly have a listing under 'Osteopaths,' or under 'Registered Osteopaths.' The initials D.O., standing for Diploma in Osteopathy, usually follow the practitioner's name on his sign or other identification. Some of the more enlightened doctors will now recommend an osteopath to you – yet he must use neuromuscular manipulation. Check with him before you go, to find out whether or not he does this technique. (Most naturopaths also specialize in the neuromuscular technique.)

I recommend osteopathic manipulation not only for those suffering from rheumatoid arthritis but for all persons who want to accelerate their cure.

## Special note on osteopathic manipulation

It is *not* a substitute for the banning of processed foods.

It is *not* a substitute for the initial diet of raw fresh fruits, raw fresh vegetables, organ meats, and fresh seafood.

It is *not* a substitute for the continuing maintenance diet aimed at keeping you arthritis-free.

It is *not* a substitute for proper elimination aimed at ridding your body of accumulated poisons.

It is *not* a substitute for your own body manipulation to create better circulation through motion and movement

It *is* an adjunct, or extra, to the arthritis cure set forth in this book.

## For your action

The delicate chemical balance in your body as you get rid of your arthritis needs to be reinforced by special attention to the best possible diet (closest to the initial diet) and the best possible elimination. Kick the aspirin habit, except when absolutely necessary to relieve pain relapse caused possibly by inclement weather. Use these motions as they apply to you to help your blood circulate:

- In bed, knees up, roll side to side.
- In bed, knees up, rock back and forth.
- In bed, toes up, let toes fall outward.
- Intone "O-m-m-m."
- Any movement that feels good.
- Wrist shake.
- Knee pendulum.
- In chair, bend back, straighten, repeat.

Next, walk farther and faster keeping a log of your accomplishment to record the improvement. Go on to swimming, bicycling, jogging or wood chopping as you improve, always below the level of fatigue.

# CHAPTER 7

# Why Certain Foods Are Your Best Medicine for Arthritis

There is good common nutritional sense why the arthritis-cure diet works. You can enjoy a wide range of delicious foods if you understand some basic facts about your body's needs. You won't learn these facts in restaurants, or reading the food advertisements, or reading the labels on packages. All you may learn there is what not to eat. This chapter expands your food horizons even beyond gourmet levels to prevent, cure, and stay cured of, crippling arthritis.

Arthritis is only one of the many threats to the health and well-being of man. When you are rid of your arthritis, your health problems may be far from over. This is because the world is getting to be less and less of a benign place to live and more and more a hostile environment.

I teach you to eat fresh fruits and fresh vegetables. But tomorrow the fruits and vegetables you buy may be almost devoid of some minerals that are essential to good health. Our present methods of farming do not fully recognize the need to replenish the soil *naturally*. As a result, the problems of adequate nutrition are growing quite complex indeed.

This chapter is intended to make you aware of what the body needs so that even long after you may have forgotten about this book, you will remember what to watch out for in guarding your health. You will remember how to keep your guard up against man's inhumane contamination of man. You will know how to keep your awareness up for sources of the best nutrition – the best foods your money can buy.

And, most important for right now, you will continue to transform that delicate chemical balance which follows the disappearance of your arthritis pain into a solid margin of safety for continued good health.

## New poisons that await us

The death by suicide of a 28-year-old woman in Japan caused a furore throughout the country. The woman had killed herself, as her diary divulged, because she suspected she had cadmium poisoning. An autopsy revealed she was right.

Cadmium is a metallic element found in zinc ores and used in metal manufacture, electro-plating and atomic fission control. It is bluish white in colour.

The girl had worked as a lathe operator in a zinc company. She had constant pain throughout her body, but the doctors failed to diagnose the trouble. Cadmium poisoning, like the poisoning that causes arthritis, goes to the bones. The cadmium deprives the bones of calcium. The bones can become so brittle that ribs snap just from coughing.

This case has alerted Japan to the dangers of cadmium and other chemicals. They have checked a number of rice fields and found unsafe concentrations of that poisonous element in a number of paddy fields as well as in vegetable samples.

It has served to dramatize the price that Japan is paying for her rapidly growing economy. It is a price that cannot be tolerated very long. All countries with industrial activity must turn part of their energies and profits back to discovering equally economic ways of controlling pollution.

Perhaps this is beginning to happen. But at the rate it is progressing, you cannot wait. You must take immediate steps towards pollution avoidance for your individual protection.

## Be your own nutritionist

To navigate a healthy course between processed foods towards naturally nutritious foods, you need to know some basic facts about proteins, fats, and carbohydrates. You also need to become more aware of the source of the food that you are about to put into your mouth.

No, I don't mean which aisle in which supermarket. I mean what state or region of the country and, if possible where local produce is concerned, whose farm.

Suppose you have read two separate stories in your local newspaper recently. One story was about farmer 'A' annoying the neighbours because his spraying with DDT may be affecting a common water supply. The other story was about farmer 'B' who was bringing in truckloads of animal manure to fertilize. This was annoying his neighbours with the odour and the flies. Whose farm stand would you prefer?

Suppose you insisted on the taste test rather than judging by news stories, what do you think the outcome of a blindfold test on tomatoes or lettuce from both farms might be?

There isn't the slightest doubt about it. The naturally fertilized soil produces far tastier food.

## General guidelines

Guidelines for arthritis-free menus are not to be found necessarily in popular magazines. These guidelines are found outdoors, in the rural locations where nature still dominates over concrete and artificial chemicals.

As much as we try to shut nature out with concrete walls, divert attention from nature with television sets, 'conquer' nature with civilized products, we remain natural living creatures – creatures of nature, responsive to nature.

Depend on nature and you have a reliable source for dietary guidance.

- A potato is best for you as nature created it – skin and all – and cooked only enough to be soft.
- Grains should be eaten whole, not broken down to component parts, or refined.
- An apple should be eaten from skin to core – as nature made it.

## Canned, frozen, and other processed foods

Of course, as you can see, this knocks down canned asparagus.* It knocks down frozen asparagus as well. It knocks down asparagus dried, powdered, or creamed, or in any as yet unthought of unnatural state.**

It leaves raw fresh asparagus as your best bet.

But it leaves two questions unanswered:

- How was it grown? (Chemicals, sprays, quality of soil?)
- How will it be processed by me?

The first of these questions is most difficult to answer in these days of mass marketing. Where farmers' markets still exist in small towns or where farm stands dot the countryside, you can find out about a farm and its practices easier than when you buy in a chain supermarket.

Organic farmers are natural farmers. They know the importance of composting soft garbage for replenishing the soil. They know the importance of adding animal manure to the compost to enrich the soil. They know the importance of earth worms in the aeration of the soil. They know the importance of mulching such as with salt hay to keep moisture in the soil and to keep weeds from robbing the soil. And they know the importance of location and rotation of crops, exploiting the affinity of one crop for another, reducing the attraction the crops have to insects and ravagers.

Why don't all farmers know and practise these methods? Simply because it costs more.

"... And produces less!" a farmer may respond in self-defence. True, in a way. But ten pounds of forced lettuce may not have the food value of five pounds of naturally grown lettuce. It may look like lettuce, feel like lettuce, even taste like lettuce; but when you eat it, your body knows the difference.

---

*   If you suffer from gout, avoid eating asparagus as it may add to your symptoms.
** More recent thinking recognizes the benefits of some frozen and canned foods. See page 7.

Your body is shortchanged.

I'm not going to try to alter our economic system by demanding that all farmers be organic farmers. But you who want to avoid arthritis, and you who are ridding yourself of its misery and want to stay rid of it, must be careful about the sources of your foods. You must at least lean in the direction away from chemical fertilizers and poison sprays whenever the availability of knowledge permits you to.

Let's get back to that asparagus. You bought it from a fine farmer. ("No, ma'am, we never have to use spray on our asparagus.") Now you are ready to prepare it for your table.

## Home-food processing

You wash it. You immerse it in water and boil away. You boil away the vitamins, dissolve most of the minerals, pour the water down the sink with all the 'good' in it.

Then you eat what's left and call it asparagus.

Again, your body is shortchanged.

Here, you are the culprit, not somebody else. But at least you are in control. All you have to do is change the way you cook. That's a lot easier than tracing the source of supermarket carrots.

We hear a lot of balanced diets. The nutritionists talk about proteins, fats, and carbohydrates. They understand what these mean to the body. They tell you what foods contain what percentages of these three basic ingredients.

One may say you must have 50 per cent carbohydrate, 25 per cent fat and 25 per cent protein to have a balanced diet. Another nutritionist may change those percentages up or down to describe a balanced diet.

Suppose you pick one and conform to his directions. Your carbohydrates are largely canned fruits, frozen (cooked) vegetables or doughnuts. Your fats are the grease in which the doughnuts and other 'goodies' are fried. Your proteins are in hamburgers, from beet shot with growth-encouraging medication and in the eggs from chickens that never see the natural light of day.

You have the perfect combination of carbohydrates, fats, and proteins. But do you have good nutrition?

Three cheers for a balanced diet. But let's not be fooled: a scale registers 'balance' with nothing on it.

## The truth about a balanced diet

We all have so much to learn about the body. We know so little about what the body needs and what it does with what it gets.

Most of the talk about a balanced diet can be translated, "Don't overdo anything. Keep on eating everything. Keep on doing what you're doing. Leave it to the body to accept what it needs. It knows better than we do."

There's a certain amount of wisdom in that. It works best when the foods we choose are raw, fresh, and unprocessed. When the balanced calories we are eating are empty of natural nutrients and full of synthetic non-nutrients, we are kidding ourselves about such a diet being balanced. If you are suffering from arthritis, or any other disease for that matter, you just cannot afford to kid yourself.

*You must be your own nutritionist.* You must know exactly what you are putting into the receiving end of your digestive canal.

### The secrets of natural food

You must get your proteins, fats, and carbohydrates, but they must be in the most natural form possible. The more unnatural they are, the more changed in molecular structure by processing or cooking, the less able the body is to cope with them, much less benefit from them. In their most natural form, you find them replete with vitamins and minerals.

These are the secrets of nature that nutritionists have discovered. There is much more to be discovered. Meanwhile, they have spotted a family or ingredients that appear to trigger good healthy minds and bodies. Some are called vitamins. Others are called by the names previously given them by biochemists. Most are now being synthesized in laboratories and manufacturing plants.

Like other efforts of man to improve on nature manufacturing creates problems. The main problem is: the body knows the difference. It uses natural vitamins and organically based minerals much more readily than the synthesized vitamins and the mined minerals. It uses natural oils, fatty acids, and many types of proteins when raw or natural but not as readily or not at all when boiled, extracted, or meddled with.

So once again, being your own nutritionist comes down to sticking as close as you can to nature.

If close to nature it is not very close where you live, then you should know about vitamin and mineral supplements. I have recommended brewers' yeast and cod liver oil. These are natural food supplements. There are others. Look for the *natural*.

But first let me give you a capsuled picture of the body you live in, what it needs, and what makes it thrive even better. There are many fine books written on this subject. Some are listed in the bibliography you will find at the end of this book. I certainly cannot do much more than list and categorize.

Be your own nutritionist. As a past or present arthritic, or if you wish to avoid being either, you have no choice.

## Vitamins – what they do for you and where to find them

"What vitamins are best for my arthritis?" I've been asked this question countless times. It's like organizing a baseball team and asking, "What position do I start with?"

You need the whole team.

All vitamins are supplied by our natural foods – naturally grown, naturally transported and stored, naturally prepared. Any one of those three factors can sound the death knell for some or all of the vitamin content of what we eat.

The body needs only minute amounts of these organic substances. Yet they play vital roles in the assimilation of nutrients and the smooth functioning of the body. Here is a summary of what they do and where they can be found.

## Types of vitamins and their sources

*Vitamin A*. Deficiency in humans can cause impairment of bone formation. Vitamin A aids all growth, provides resistance to infection, prolongs vitality. *Best foods*: Greens, such as mustard, turnip and dandelion; squash, kale, broccoli; calf's liver.

*Vitamin B$_1$*. Also called thiamine, a lack of it can cause loss of muscle tone, irritability, fatigue, constipation – all to be avoided especially by arthritics. *Best foods*: Brewers' yeast, seeds, beef heart, beef kidney, oysters, free-range eggs. Thiamine is easily destroyed during cooking.*

*Vitamin B$_2$*. Also called riboflavin, a lack of it can cause nervous depression, dermatitis, eye problems. It is especially beneficial to the soft tissues of the body, including muscles. *Best foods*: Some greens and other vegetables containing vitamin A plus brewers' yeast, raw milk, and organ meats (kidneys, liver, sweetbreads).

*Vitamin B$_3$*. Called niacin. Symptoms of deficiency include depression and memory loss. Good food sources include rice bran, fresh tuna fish, chicken liver, and brown rice.

*Vitamin B$_5$*. Called pantothenic acid and a benefit to healthy liver functioning as well as to the brain and nervous system. *Best foods*: Fish, poultry, lean meats, liver, brewers' yeast.

*Vitamin B$_6$*. Called pyridoxine, this is a nerve-muscle vitamin, helpful in disorders such as muscular dystrophy It is certainly important to arthritics on the mend. *Best foods*: Fresh leafy vegetables, wheatgerm, bananas, most meats, especially turkey and liver.

*Vitamin B$_{12}$*. An animal-protein factor essential for forming bone marrow and important to the central nervous system. *Best foods*: Liver, meat, eggs, milk.

*Vitamin C*. Popularly known as ascorbic acid and frequently used in massive doses to combat colds and infections. It is used by the body to produce *collagen*, a protein needed in bone, skin, and supportive tissue. *Best foods*: Rose hips, green peppers, cabbage,

---

* All of the B vitamins are damaged by heat, and foods rich in these nutrients should be eaten raw whenever possible.

tomatoes, brussels sprouts, cauliflower, broccoli, strawberries, watermelon cantaloupe.

*Vitamin D.* Very important to the cure and prevention of arthritis because without it the body cannot properly absorb calcium and phosphorus from foods, both needed in bone growth. *Best foods*: Cod liver oil, eggs, milk, sunflower seeds.

*Vitamin E.* An aid to liver functioning. Promotes radiant skin, hair. *Best foods*: Vegetable oils of corn and soy; leafy vegetables like spinach; eggs, seeds, meat.

*Unsaturated fatty acids.* They help the body utilize other vitamins. A factor in the distribution of calcium throughout the body. *Best foods*: Salad oils like peanut, safflower, soy, and sunflower.

*Vitamin K.* Helps the liver form prothrombin, a factor in blood clotting. A longevity agent. *Best foods*: Fresh green, leafy vegetables, tomatoes, egg yolk, liver.

*Bioflavonoids.* These natural plant compounds work with other vitamins and minerals to maintain blood-vessel walls and the tiny veins and capillaries in good working order. Closely associated with vitamin C. *Best foods*: Apples, lettuce, cabbage, green peppers, spinach, parsley, watercress.

## Other sources and powers of vitamins

Notice how some foods appear again and again as best sources – fresh leafy vegetables, green peppers, liver. This is one of the reasons why these foods are on the arthritis-cure diet.

Some foods stand out as vitamin sources. A veritable treasury of vitamins and minerals, for instance, is the sunflower seed. It has significant quantities of vitamins B, $B_1$, $B_2$, D, and E, with such important minerals as phosphorus, potassium, magnesium, and a few more to boot.

Other standouts are familiar to you as they are on your arthritis-cure diet – brewers' yeast, cod liver oil, liver, and other organ meats.

**A case of scurvy due to malnutrition**

A middle-aged banker went to his doctor complaining of pains in his arms and legs. He was constantly tired, had frequent headaches and rashes. The doctor could find nothing wrong and referred him to a surgeon. The surgeon was equally baffled and sent him to a neurologist whose battery of tests failed to turn up any clue. The case was reported in an issue of a nutrition magazine and here is what was discovered.

The man was a widower who was fixing his own food – the usual quickie breakfasts, hamburger lunches, and martini and steak dinners. No fruits. No vegetables.

He had scurvy.

Nobody who examined him dreamt that a banker could be suffering from malnutrition. In our society today, however, it is less a question of affluence than it is a knowledge of natural foods.

## Supplements of foods

If you take these natural foods and if you do not destroy vitamins by cooking, eating as many vegetables raw as possible, you need not be concerned about buying vitamin supplements. Those who do feel that additional vitamins are needed should lean toward the naturally produced vitamins as opposed to synthetic types.

Don't attempt to exceed recommended doses on the premise that if a little is good, a lot is better. Although most vitamins and minerals are non-toxic and will be eliminated when excess amounts are consumed, still there is some evidence pointing to an immunity mechanism being activated. In other words, you may have to continue to overdose yourself to absorb just minimum amounts.

Certainly there's no point in getting into that condition. The late Dr Norman Jolliffe, founder of the first anticoronary club, found low levels of vitamin A in patients with rheumatoid arthritis. He often prescribed doses of vitamin A several times the 5,000 international units recommended by the Natural Research Council. If in doubt about vitamin doses ask your doctor or naturopath.

In a way I'm sorry vitamins were discovered a few decades ago. Now we give the alphabet the credit instead of the fresh, green leafy vegetables or the calf's liver or the raw milk. That's where the respect belongs. We need to be devoted to these farm foods, not to bottles on a shelf.

We need to taste the difference between depleted foods and living foods. We need to re-educate our taste buds so that our likes shift from soggy hamburgers, greasy french fries, and sweet cake, candy, and cokes to crispy raw garden fresh delights, lusty meats, and sun-ripened raw fruits.

## Minerals that conquer arthritis

I want to talk for a minute to you who have had arthritis for a long time and who have had to live with bone enlargement and joint impairment. You can experience a return towards normal bone structure simply by being rigorously faithful to the diet, elimination, and movement instructions I have given you.

Faithful to the treatment was Mr F. B. Perhaps the incentive to regain your health at 35 is greater than in later years. It certainly is a young age to be suffering from general arthritis. It was most severe in the hip joints. He walked with extreme pain and only with the aid of a cane. He could not turn in bed. He had to sleep on his back and then only with heavy sedation.

He was ready to eat anything – even raw fresh fruits, raw fresh vegetables, and raw liver. In a week he was sleeping like a baby and walking like a man. But, mind you, those hips still had a long way to go.

He was so pleased with the improvement that rather than add new foods rapidly he strove to consolidate his gains. He added a few, but felt his way slowly with them. It paid off. He found that bones can respond to a dietary respect for nature and the human body.

Six months later, there was decided improvement. Bony proliferation had been partially absorbed, creating greater joint space and ease of mobility.

I'm not going to pretend to know just what vitamins and minerals in what proportions are ideal for the cure of arthritis. Even if it were possible to assemble such information from controlled nutrition, which it isn't, I am sure that the results would vary for different people and different types of arthritis.

Play it safe. Eat all vitamins and minerals recommended in this book. Or as the nutritionists say, "Eat a balanced diet." Only don't let me see you with any cans or boxes or jars in your hand!

## Diet minerals for health

Here is the mineral information in basic, simplified form:

*Calcium*. The key mineral in arthritis, often lacking in arthritis sufferers because some foods like white bread and some drugs like DDT interfere with its absorption. *Best foods*: Blackstrap molasses, green vegetables, seafood, free-range chickens (not raised all their lives in chicken houses).

*Iron*. Helps the blood carry oxygen to the cells and remove carbon dioxide. *Best foods*: Blackstrap molasses, leafy green vegetables, liver, free-range egg yolks.

*Phosphorus*. Important to proper functioning of nerves, glands, muscles. Works closely with calcium. *Best foods*: Meats, fish, cheese, free-range chickens, and eggs.

*Manganese*. Activates enzymes to aid the tissues. Only traces are needed. *Best foods*: Green vegetables, especially when grown in organically enriched soil.

*Copper*. Aids in the body's use of vitamin C and iron. *Best foods*: Huckleberries, blackstrap molasses, liver, leafy green vegetables.

*Potassium*. Aids in proper digestive elimination. Feeds the nerves, the heart, the muscles. *Best foods*: Green leafy vegetables, tomatoes, carrots, cucumbers, apple cider vinegar, cranberries, and most fruits and berries.

*Iodine*. A regulator of the body's rate of metabolism via the thyroid gland. Just traces needed. *Best foods*: Ocean fish, shellfish.

Again – an overlap in many of the sources for these minerals and in the sources of vitamins and minerals.

Modern research indicates that there are other minerals we should consume as part of our diet, or in food supplements. These are:

*Boron* – Research suggests this mineral is important in maintaining healthy bone density.

*Copper* – Research shows that low levels of dietary copper may inhibit normal bone growth, and contribute to brittle bones.

*Manganese* – Needed to maintain bone density.

*Selenium* – A powerful antioxidant that works with vitamins C and E to reduce the ageing effects of free radicals, selenium also plays a vital role in the production of anti-inflammatory prostaglandins (hormone-like substances in the blood). It is also vital for a healthy heart and liver.

*Zinc* – A component of many vital metabolic process in the body, zinc is needed for normal tissue growth and to fight infection.

## A generous list of the best foods you can eat

As you add foods to the first week's diet, choose from the *Best foods* cited above as sources for both vitamins and nutrients. Do you consider this limiting?

You had better take another look. The sources of these health-giving nutrients are practically limitless.

Here is a surprising list of these best foods in various categories.

You can have three banquets a day with them, every day different for months.

## Your most valuable foods

*Vegetables*

| | |
|---|---|
| Carrots | Swiss chard |
| Peas* | Kohlrabi |
| Black-eyed peas* | Tomatoes |
| Green peppers | Beet tops |
| Lentils* | Radishes |
| Pole (green) beans | Parsnips |

| | |
|---|---|
| Butter beans* | Cauliflowers |
| Mung beans | Swede |
| Aduki beans | Turnips |
| Runner beans | Aubergine |
| Chickpeas* | Broccoli |
| Corn | Brussels sprouts |
| Cucumbers | Parsley |
| Marrow | Salsify |
| Red cabbage | Asparagus* |
| Savoy cabbage | Onions |
| Spinach* | Spring onions |
| Kale | Leek |
| Mushrooms | Chives |
| Horseradish | Okra |
| Brown rice | Lettuce |
| Wild rice | Watercress |
| Millet | Escarole |
| Buckwheat | Beetroot |
| | Endive |

### Fowl (free range)

| | |
|---|---|
| Chicken | Turkey |
| Duck | Squab |
| Goose | |

### Meats (Beef)

| | |
|---|---|
| Roasts (all kinds) | Steaks (all kinds) |
| Shank meat | Short ribs |
| Chopped beef | Flank |
| Stew beef | |

* People suffering from gout should avoid pulses rich in purines. They should also avoid asparagus.

### Meats (Lamb)

| | |
|---|---|
| Roast leg of lamb | Lamb patties |
| Lamb shank | Lamb stew |
| Chops (all kinds) | |

### Meats (Pork)

| | |
|---|---|
| Roasts (all kinds) | Pigs knuckles |
| Chops (all kinds) | Spare ribs |

### Meats (Veal)

| | |
|---|---|
| Chops | Veal roast |
| Cutlets (not breaded) | Breast of veal |

### Meats (Organ)

| | |
|---|---|
| Liver | Heart |
| Kidney | Tripe (cattle only) |
| Sweetbreads** | Brains** |

### Seafood

| | |
|---|---|
| Striped bass | Halibut |
| Cod | Tuna (fresh) |
| Sole | Whiting |
| Scallops (bay)* | Sea bass |
| Scallops (deep sea)* | Fluke |
| Lobster* | Smelts |
| Shrimp* | Salmon (fresh) |
| Crabs (soft shell)* | Clams |
| Crabs (hard)* | Mussels |
| Red snapper | Oysters |
| Eels | Herring (boned)* |
| Pomfret | Fish roe* |

\* Gout sufferers should avoid all shellfish and crustaceans. Both herring and roe (fish eggs) are high in purines that can trigger an attack of gout.

\*\* Because of the risks involved with potentially contracting BSE from certain organ meats, it is advisable to only purchase these meats from reputable suppliers.

### Fruits

| | |
|---|---|
| Golden apples | Mulberries |
| Red apples | Rhubarb |
| Northern Spy apples | Currants |
| Rome apples | Figs |
| Baldwin apples | Prunes |
| Russets | Plums |
| Bananas | Nectarines |
| Blueberries | Peaches |
| Blackberries | Bartlett pears |
| Raspberries | Apricots |
| Strawberries | Cherries |
| Gooseberries | Grapes (all varieties) |
| Loganberries | Melons (all varieties) |

### Nuts

| | |
|---|---|
| Hazel nuts | Peanuts |
| Walnuts | Chestnuts |
| Brazil nuts | Pistachio nuts |
| Almonds | Pine kernels |
| Pecans | Cashews |

### Seeds

| | |
|---|---|
| Pumpkin | Linseed |
| Alfalfa | Butter beans |
| Aduki beans | Haricot beans |
| Sesame | |

### Other food exceptions and additions

I have not listed *eggs*, because as you know the usual poultry-farm eggs are quite diminished in nutritional value compared to the eggs of their pecking cousins. I use the term free-range eggs to denote the natural variety. If you can get organic free-range eggs from chickens not cooped up in 'chicken farms' they belong on the list.

Do you want to know what the *most nutritious cheeses are*? I'll tell you but it won't do you much good as you'll probably never find any:

Cheese made from the spring milk of either goats, sheep, or cows.

*Tofu* This is fermented soya-bean curd, often used in Chinese cooking, and is an excellent source of protein as an alternative to cheese, eggs, and meat. It is tasteless but can be used in a variety of ways in casseroles, dressings, and desserts, if flavoured with herbs, yeast extracts, or natural juices.

When you plan for meals with maximum punch, *Tahini* is another food that is packed with flavour and high in nutrients. Made of crushed sesame seeds, it can be added to dressings, dips, and sauces.

## The essential food categories

The food we eat becomes our body. The air we breathe supplies an important ingredient – oxygen. We get no nourishment, no energy, no tissue- or bone-building material from anything except the food we eat.

If you are to be your own nutritionist, you should know that all food is made up of three major categories – protein, fat, and carbohydrates. Don't choose among them. All three are necessary to a healthy, arthritis-free body.

Let's take a quick look at each.

### Proteins

The word 'protein' means 'primary'. It is the very fabric of our bodies – our tissues, muscles, organs, blood, etc. Proteins are composed largely of amino acids. There are supposed to be at least 32 of these amino acids. The body can manufacture most of these in its own laboratory, or digestive system, but, it must have proteins to start with.

There are eight (some authorities say ten) amino acids that the body cannot make. They have to be supplied by some outside source. These are called *essential* amino acids simply because the body cannot make them, not that they are any more essential to the body than the other amino acids.

We cannot exist without proteins. All our body cells contain proteins. So, we must get our proteins daily. In that protein intake, we must be especially sure to get the eight or ten essential amino acids.

Here are some signs of protein deficiency in order of appearance:

a. General sluggishness, early fatigue, lack of energy.
b. Abdominal distention, constipation, and dilation of the bowel.
c. Generalized swelling or an appearance of increased weight.

These symptoms become progressively worse as the deficiency deepens and more symptoms are added, particularly noticeable in arthritis.

A protein must be complete in order to be of full value to the body. It must contain the essential amino acids. Animal proteins are more likely to contain these essential amino acids in adequate amounts than are vegetable proteins.

*Best protein foods*: Organic milk, fish, liver, kidneys, muscle meats, eggs, brewers' yeast, soybean products.

Vegetarians should use soya products, such as tofu, cheese, and eggs, as protein sources. If you have problems tolerating cows' milk use soya milk or tofu as an alternative to milk and cheese. Essential amino acids can be obtained by combining one-part pulses with two-parts grains, such as brown rice or millet.

## Fats

Here again there are the animal fats and the vegetable variety we more commonly know as oils.

Oil is very important to people suffering from arthritis.

If you have arthritis, you may be suffering from an oil deficiency. But you are very likely to be suffering also from a deficiency of other nutrients, – and from a deficiency in the eliminating department, especially the elimination from the body of chemicals, sprays, additives, colourings, preservatives, and the like.

## The health case for eating fats

Fat needs a public-relations man! It has acquired a bad image. One reason is it is assumed that if you eat fat you become fat – fat and ugly. This has been supported by the fact that there are more calories in an ounce of oil and fat than in an ounce of carbohydrate or an ounce of protein. But what we forget is that there are two factors not taken into account by merely equating an ounce of each to the calories in that ounce:

1 It takes more energy (calories) to digest fats and proteins than it does carbohydrates.
2 Proteins and fats tend to increase the body's rate of metabolism, while carbohydrates tend to slow it down.

This is not meant to be a defence for fat and I have no intention of being its public-relations mentor, but it is important in the whole nutrition picture and whatever 'black-eye' fat may have with you, give it its nutritional due.

Then there's this matter of hard fats, soft fats; of animal fats versus vegetable fats; of the saturated and the polyunsaturated. What's a fellow to do?

## The whole diet

If we look to nature – a more reliable source is hard to find, even in the university food and nutrition departments – we find that there are other carnivorous and herbivorous creatures faced with the same problem. Like the racoon.

He takes his fat as he get it. He eats nuts, fruit, mice, whole fat and all. He even eats a whole fish, when he can. If man doesn't shoot him, he lives a healthy, happy, and long life. No arthritis. No disease. No one presses out corn to get corn oil for him. He gets his corn oil right in the kernel, together with the other nutrients associated with the whole kernel.

The racoon does the same with his wheat. When he finds a wheat field, he eats the whole wheat kernel. He doesn't have someone press out the oil of the wheat so he can have his wheatgerm oil. He enjoys his wheat with all the nutrient factors intact. He doesn't get high blood-cholesterol levels, hardening of the arteries, coronary attacks, or even strokes for that matter. He just lives a happy and healthy life. No illnesses, no doctors, no dentists.

The chemist is trained to synthesize. When he successfully creates a faithful replica of a given molecule he is satisfied that he has a product that is as good as the original and that the human body will accept it as readily as it does the original. When he has successfully completed synthesizing all we need from A to Z, he assumes that we will readily accept A through Z.

But we accept what we have traditionally accepted. It goes way back to the millenniums of our evolution. Examine the foetus as it grows from fertilized egg and you see these ages of evolution telescoped into days and weeks. Every one of these ages is evident.

*There is no substitute for natural evolution.*

Fat is necessary in our diet. What is the best way to get it? As we did while evolving.

We have always obtained our fats in natural ways, combined with other nutrients. We are built to accept and use fats most expeditiously when contained in animals and plants, meats and vegetables.

### Best foods for healthy fats

Oily fish (for example mackerel, fresh tuna, salmon, and herring), nuts, seeds, and green leafy foods are your best sources of the healthy fats needed to control the damage and pain caused by arthritis. These foods are rich in essential fatty acids, about which more is said later. (See pages 203–05.) Because these fats are found in small amounts in food, supplement your diet with cod liver oil or fish oil. (Scientific evidence shows that two or three meals a week containing oily fish also helps maintain a healthy heart and cardiovascular system.)

### Carbohydrates

These are the easiest to come by. They provide fuel for the body.

They are in all fruits, grains, vegetables, nuts, seeds – even meats, fish, and eggs have a trace.

What do Eskimos do about carbohydrates on a diet of polar bear or seal blubber? The body cannot manufacture protein but it can manufacture fat and carbohydrate from protein. And it can manufacture carbohydrate from fat. Protein is the only one of the three that the body cannot produce.

The overweight person is quite familiar with this ability of the body. He sees the fat accumulate in his body from too many sweets and starches. Then he eliminates these sweets and starches, and sees his body convert the fat on him into carbohydrate that is then burned for energy.

### Best foods for carbohydrates

Fruits, vegetables, brown rice, seeds, nuts.

Get your carbohydrates from *natural* foods. They contain a great many other nutrient factors as nature intended.

If you get your carbohydrates from refined foods, such as refined cane sugar in cakes, cookies, ice cream, candy, jams, jellies, and marmalade, and from other man-made foods such as macaroni and spaghetti, little to no other food factors are present.

Then things start to go wrong. One example: This puts a severe burden on the pancreas. If vitamin $B_6$ isn't present in the refined foods, and most often it isn't, pyruvic acid cannot be broken down. The presence of this acid causes fatigue and disturbance to nerve trunks or nerve impulses along those trunks, causing nerve irritability and nerve degeneration. I could list 100 other serious malfunctions, most of them interrelated and all the direct result of refined, empty calories.

To get the most out of life and the best of health, obtain your carbohydrates *only* from natural foods.

If you have arthritis, these refined foods are absolutely forbidden.

## Ten commandments for arthritis-free dining

Let me sum up this technical, and often boring subject by giving you ten basic rules to follow in being your own arthritis-free nutritionist:

1 Balance your menu fairly evenly between proteins, fats, and carbohydrates. A few percentage points up or down is not significant.

2 Eat some raw fruit or raw vegetable every meal.

3 Avoid high heat methods that can alter food structure and destroy nutrients. Frying with very low heat in just enough butter or kidney-beef suet to prevent sticking is definitely permissible.

4 Cook food as little as possible.

5 Save pot liquor produced in cooking, for soups, gravies, and juice drinks.

6 Favour organ meats over flesh and muscle meats.

7 Use bones for marrowbone soup.

8 Favour the whole natural food, such as grain, over parts or extracts; eat the skin or outer covering, where edible, not just the inside.

9 Favour organic or natural sources of all meat and produce.

10 Avoid entirely all flour and flour products; refined sugar; artificial sweeteners; frozen fruits. Citrus fruits should be avoided in the beginning when the joints are hot, swollen, and painful. Later they may be tried. Avoid jams, jellies, marmalades; all canned or otherwise preserved foods; all prepared, semi-prepared, refined or manufactured foods, cola, carbonated beverages, beer, wine, liquor, tea, coffee, candy, ice cream, and other sweets.

## For your action

You become your own best nutritionist when you understand the meaning of the word natural. Once you do, you avoid the synthetic. You steer clear of chemicals and additives and refined products.

- Learn the vocabulary of natural nutrition – vitamins, minerals, proteins, fats, carbohydrates.
- Make a copy of the *best foods* for each and post them in your kitchen, along with the list of *YOUR MOST VALUABLE FOODS*.
- Check every food before you eat it to make sure that it, or a close natural relative, is on that list.

# CHAPTER 8

# Selected Recipes for Food Enjoyment in Arthritis-free Living

Here are many recipes for delicious soups, salads, entrees, blended juices, and desserts with emphasis on your most valuable living foods. Many of these recipes are permissible during your first days with the arthritis cure. Others had better wait until the pain, heat, and swelling have subsided. Devise, revise, alter, and adapt. There is a world of natural, unprocessed, nutritious food to enjoy in your arthritis-free living from now on.

So strong are the vested interests in drugs and in sugar and flour products that they have succeeded in making it illegal in some parts of the United States for anyone except a doctor to state in public that diet or nutrition has something to do with health or the cure of disease.

They are reported to have pressured the US Food and Drug Administration to propose regulations prohibiting the identification of foods or food supplements as being natural or organically grown as opposed to synthetic or grown with chemical fertilizers.

Can you imagine what would happen to food supplies if the US government continued to represent not the consumer but the manufacturers who place profit above nutrition? Or what would happen to health care and disease prevention if medical doctors were allowed a monopoly, and treatment by palliative drugs was all that was available to those suffering from arthritis and other similar diseases?

Fortunately, thanks to growing consumer vigilance and awareness, freedom to advertise natural produce and advocate its use for health care is permitting the health-conscious person to take steps to avoid pollution of his body.

## Your basic steps

Your steps are largely in the supermarket and in your kitchen.

Buy fresh fruits and fresh vegetables from sources you know are the least contaminated by fertilizers and pesticides. Choose organic produce wherever possible. If you must buy non-organic produce, wash all leafy vegetables well in a mild vinegar solution to loosen surface film. Peel other foods: that includes apples, pears, potatoes, carrots, swedes, and anything else that may be contaminated with agro-chemicals. Buy organ meats. Then enlarge your shopping list only as your steps are pain-free and your body no longer pained by arthritis.

In the kitchen, you can take steps to utilize foods in their *natural* nutritional form.

If you were a vitamin or a mineral, can you imagine what would be left of you if you were immersed in scalding fat or baked, boiled, broiled, seared, simmered, stewed, sizzled, roasted, and barbecued?

We must cook many of our foods in order for us to find them palatable and enjoyable. Yet some schools of natural nutrition advocate eating more than 50 per cent of our daily food intake in a raw or uncooked state. This is a fine goal to shoot for. When you hit a target like that you are boosting your level of nutrition to a point where friends are bound to comment on your youthful radiance, and dentists and doctors wonder why they no longer see you.

## Healthy food preparation

- If food must be cooked, use as little water as possible to cook it.
- If food must be cooked, use as low a temperature as possible to cook it.
- If food must be cooked, keep it on or in the heat the minimum time necessary to cook it.

Above are the three axioms for nutritious cookery and they have special application to arthritis cure. Let's take a closer look at the elements of each axiom.

Walk into most kitchens just before dinner time and you'll see vegetables cooking in a pot on the stove, drowning in water that usually at least half submerges them – and half ruins them. All you really need to cook vegetables is enough water so that some will remain after boiling. Most vitamins and minerals are water soluble. That means that while the cabbage itself might be there, its nutritive essence is largely diminished, dissolved in the cooking water.

Save even the little cooking water you have left. It is valuable food! Your body needs that cooking water. If you don't feel like drinking it right there on the spot, put it in a covered jar and refrigerate it until you are ready to use it in a mixed vegetable juice, soup, stew, or sauce.

Many vegetables can be cooked without any water at all. Baking is the secret. You lose nothing down the drain. You can bake broccoli, squash, cauliflower, aubergine, just about any vegetable but preferably the root or solid type as opposed to the more delicate leafy types.

Before baking add a little butter or oil. Cover the pot. Adjust oven to a moderate temperature, surely no more than 170°C, Gas mark 3, 325°F. Check in a few minutes for tenderness. Some vegetables can take as long as 30 minutes by this method. But they cook in their own juices, and you can taste the difference.

Think in terms of low temperature no matter by what method you cook. Even meats can be largely destroyed nutritionally speaking by intense heat.

Except for barbecuing, frying puts food in closest contact with the flame or with the red-hot cooking elements. It is therefore the most destructive method of cooking. Sauté instead. As you know, that's like frying at a lower temperature.

Orientals use the *wok*, a curved bowl-like cooking utensil that raises the food slightly off the heat source. It is not designed to be very practical on electric heating elements but it works fine on gas and is a more healthful way of cooking meat or vegetables or combinations – in their own juices. (Woks are now available with a built-in electric element which makes them easy to use provided you have access to a power point.)

If you use pressure cookers, aim for using as little water as you can get away with and as little cooking time.

The proper use of microwave cooking cuts time in the kitchen and, scientific research reveals, does less damage to many nutrients than other forms of heating food. Using fresh foods, avoid processed and packaged products, and enjoy the benefits of this modern appliance.

### Benefits of 'cooking it rare'

Of course, the less time something is cooking the better for health's sake. "Hey, mum, the peas ain't done." How often the cook in the family is berated for not creating something more soft and mushy. Hit back. Get your family to know that the crisper taste of slightly cooked foods is the taste of super-health, and particularly for the sake of the arthritic.

Rare meat is more nutritious than charcoal-blackened meat. If smaller cuts of meat are used, you do not have to cook as long. Why roast the good right out of a piece of meat just to have the heat penetrate to the centre?

## The arthritis-free world of no-cook cookery

You can 'cook up' a banquet without going near the stove.

Cold soups, salads, blended nectars, and fruit desserts contain nature's bounty at its original zesty best.

All you really need is a sharp knife to slice and grate with. Toss away that peeler. The peels that are edible – as on potatoes, cucumbers, squash – contain most of the nutrients.

Juices and blenders are useful kitchen aids. The blender grinds and mixes to create a smooth consistency. The juicer does this, too, but also can be used to separate liquid from bulk. This has the advantage of getting large amounts of essence from such seemingly dry vegetables as carrots and celery, while straining out the bulk. Nevertheless, I question whether the bulk is not just as important.

Many of the recipes that follow in this chapter give you ideas for the use of a juicer or blender. One of my friends occasionally throws an ice-cream party. He serves delicious banana ice cream, pineapple sherbet, and other flavours. If you were invited you could enjoy several portions, because I know how he makes them: the fruit is skinned and frozen. Then it is put through a juicer. Nothing else. That creamy banana ice cream is nothing but pure frozen banana.

Use raw foods. Let your imagination be your Cordon Bleu. Slice and grate. Mix and arrange. Enjoy crisp natural flavours. But better yet, treat your body to their powerful arthritis-dissolving health-building nutrients.

## How you can have a health garden in your kitchen

Remember the days when people grew mushrooms in their basement? And watercress on sponges in their kitchen?

Those days may be returning as prices go up and unsprayed, unprocessed foods get harder to find.

People are now sprouting a variety of edibles. They take little space, and no time because you eat the sprouts. Here are some foods you can sprout in two to four days:

| | | |
|---|---|---|
| Raw peas | Mung beans | Lettuce seeds |
| Alfalfa | Raw peanuts | Clover seeds |
| Lentils | Radish seeds | Sunflower seeds |
| Soy beans | Navy beans | Pumpkin seeds |
| Almonds | Chili beans | Squash seeds |

Here is how it is done. First, soak the seeds in water about 12 to 15 hours. Then drain, rinse, and put in an open jar. Cover jar with a porous material like cheesecloth, fasten with a rubber band and tilt jar downward to drain. Once a day, rinse.

Sprouts are bursting with life! They are often three or four times as nutritious as the seed or bean from which they have just emerged. This is a miracle of photosynthesis, the secret of growth of all plant life.

Use sprouts in salads, soups, or stews. Cook them alone as a vegetable, – low heat, of course.

Just looking at the miracle in your kitchen will serve to remind you that you, too, are a creature of nature, dependent not on the factories and processors for food, but on nature's sunlight, fresh air, pure water, and growing things.

## Recipes to inspire your own culinary creativity

The following recipes are from the files of my own kitchen and the kitchens of my health-minded friends. Try them. But better yet, create your own favourite dish from nutritious foods.

The asterisk (*) indicates it is a suitable recipe for your initial days following the fast you undertook to begin curing arthritis.

A small 't' indicates a teaspoon. A capital T indicates a tablespoon.

When we speak of chickens we mean free range chickens – chickens that are out grazing in the fields – not cooped up in windowless barracks for mass production for poundage only.

All recipes for four servings unless otherwise noted:

## Soups and blended mixtures

### Gazpacho*

| | |
|---|---|
| ³/₄ cup tomato juice (fresh) | 2 T olive oil |
| 1 small cucumber, coarsely cut | 2 T cider vinegar |
| 3 tomatoes, peeled | 1 clove garlic |
| ¹/₂ green pepper, seeded | 2 green onions or shallots |

Puree in blender only until chopped fine. Chill. Garnish with slices of cucumber, green pepper or chives.

## Puree of pea soup *

| | |
|---|---|
| 3 cups homemade broth or soup stock | Pinch of thyme |
| 2 cups fresh peas | 1 shallot |
| 1 avocado | (or) 1 green onion |
| 1 tomato | salt and pepper |

Cut up vegetables, blend with peas in broth. Season and heat slightly. Garnish with parsley and serve.

## Vichyssoise

| | |
|---|---|
| 1 small onion | 1 t curry powder |
| (or) 2 leeks (white parts) | (or) turmeric |
| 3 medium potatoes, sliced | 1 cup milk |
| 2 cups chicken stock (homemade) | 1 cup cream or yogurt |
| 1 T butter | Salt and pepper |

Brown onion lightly in butter. Add stock, potatoes and seasoning. Cook until tender. Puree in blender or put through sieve. Return to pan and heat to serving temperature. Or chill and garnish with chives.

## Soybean soup

| | |
|---|---|
| 1 cup soybeans | $1/2$ t salt |
| 2 whole green onions, sliced | $1/4$ t pepper |
| 2 stalks celery, sliced | $1/4$ t fresh ginger |
| 4 cups water | $1/4$ t thyme (or) fines herbes |

Soak beans for 24 hours, changing the water at least twice, and drain. Put beans in a pot with celery and water. Cook until tender (about 4 hours), then puree them (put through a strainer). Brown onion in butter, add pureed beans and seasonings. Heat. Can be garnished with sliced hard-boiled egg.

## Chinese celery soup

1¹/₂ cups coarsely chopped
   Chinese celery
4 cups homemade broth
Several slices of liver, finely sliced

¹/₂ t caraway seeds
salt and pepper to taste

Simmer about ¹/₂ hour. Add cabbage about 5 minutes before serving.

## Guacamole*

1 large ripe avocado
1 garlic clove, mashed
2 t vinegar

¹/₂ medium onion chopped
   (or) 2 green onions
¹/₂ t oregano
salt and pepper to taste

Pit avocado and mash by hand. Add all other ingredients and mix thoroughly. Or else blend in blender. Place in bowl and cover with thin layer of mayonnaise to keep from darkening. Serve as salad, relish or as snack wrapped in lettuce leaves. When used as a dip, serve with pieces of carrots sliced into strips, broken bits of raw cauliflower, raw green beans, and cherry tomatoes.

## Tofu dressing or dip

Half to whole block tofu
   (200-300g)
Half cup vegetable oil
1 T tamari or soya sauce

¹/₃ cup lemon juice
1 T tahini
Fresh mint leaves

Place the ingredients in a blender or bowl and chop or break in the mint leaves. Blend or whisk to a thick creamy consistency.

## Andalusian soup*

| | |
|---|---|
| 1 cucumber | 1 T vinegar |
| 1 green pepper, seeded | 2 T olive oil |
| 3 or 4 tomatoes | Salt and pepper to taste |
| 1 clove garlic | |

Place all ingredients in a blender with a little cold water. Blend quickly and serve very cold. Garnish with a dash of paprika.

## Fruit nog (for 2)*

| | |
|---|---|
| 1 fresh apricot, pitted | 1 cup of milk |
| (or) 1 banana, fresh peach, | 1 egg |
| fresh berries or fresh | 1 T honey |
| pineapple | |

Blend all together until smooth. Serve chilled.

## Blender mayonnaise*

| | |
|---|---|
| 1 organic free-range egg | |
| 2 T cider vinegar | Salt and freshly ground pepper |
| fresh ginger (small piece put | to taste |
| through press) | 1 cup oil (can be half olive and |
| clove garlic, pressed | half soy, peanut or other oil) |
| pinch of basil, marjoram or thyme | |

Place all ingredients but the oil into container and blend at medium speed for about 15 seconds. With the motor running, pour the oil in slowly. Blend until thickened. Refrigerate at once.

## Fish dishes

### California seafood

| | |
|---|---|
| $^1/_2$ ripe avocado per person | 1 ripe tomato, quartered |
| 2 cups crabmeat, lobster, or shrimp (cooked) | 4 T oil |
| | 2 t cider vinegar |
| $^1/_2$ medium green pepper, seeded and cut into 8ths | 1 garlic clove |
| | $^1/_2$ cup green onions (or) sliced celery |

Cut avocado lengthwise, scrape out the insides. Toss seafood with oil and vinegar. Put a small garlic clove through press for its juice. Mix with all other ingredients and fill avocado shells.

*Note:* People with gout should avoid shellfish and crustaceans, such as lobsters, crabs, and shrimp.

### Filet Mornay

| | |
|---|---|
| 2 T butter | pinch of basil, paprika |
| filets of halibut or similar fish | 1 cup yogurt |
| salt and pepper to taste | $^1/_2$ cup grated natural cheese |
| 1 sprig parsley, chopped fine | 1 T vinegar |

Butter a pan well, season and mask it with yogurt. Cover with grated cheese. Dot with butter and sprinkle with a little more paprika. Put it in the oven. After it begins to cook, add 1 T vinegar. Cook at 180°C, Gas mark 4, 350°F for about 20 minutes.

### Tahitian raw fish*

| | |
|---|---|
| 2 lbs fish (halibut, tuna or bass) | 2 stalks celery (or watercress) finely sliced |
| 4 T cider vinegar | |
| 3 tomatoes, finely sliced | salt and pepper to taste |
| 3 stalks green onions, finely chopped | 3 eggs sliced (hard-boiled or poached) |
| 1 green pepper, seeded and finely sliced | lettuce |

Cut fish into $^{1}/_{2}$ to 1-inch pieces (slightly freezing the fish makes it easier to slice finely). Marinate it in vinegar for several hours or overnight. Remove excess liquid. Arrange on bed of lettuce. Garnish with all other ingredients and serve chilled.

## Oven-broiled fish

Halve haddock, cod, halibut, salmon, or mackerel filleted. Salt and pepper to taste. Cover entire fillet with oil. Place skin side down on a greased (oil or butter) pan. Sprinkle it with paprika. Add about 2 T water or vinegar to the pan and broil until done (about 10 minutes). Do not turn. Pour over some melted butter. Garnish with parsley or watercress and serve.

## French-baked fish

| | |
|---|---|
| 1 large or several small fish | Salt and pepper to taste |
| 1 cup yogurt | Parsley, chopped |
| 1$^{1}/_{2}$ cup cider | 1 onion, sliced |

Have heads and tails removed from fish (allow 1 per person if small). Place in a pan and cover with cider. Bake in moderate oven for about 15 minutes. Mix yogurt with the remaining cider in a pan and garnish with parsley and serve.

## Poultry

## Hawaiian chicken curry

| | |
|---|---|
| 1 small carrot | 2 T curry powder |
| 1 stewing chicken, cut in joints | Salt and pepper to taste |
| 2 T butter or oil | 2 cups of hot water |
| 2 medium onions, finely chopped | 2 egg yolks beaten in |
| $^{1}/_{2}$ t dried ginger | $^{1}/_{2}$ cup cream |

Brown chicken pieces in butter or oil in skillet. Remove to pan and cover with water, add carrot and simmer, covered, until tender.

Meanwhile, brown onions slightly in butter remaining in skillet. Stir in seasonings. Take out chicken and remove skin. Add onions and seasonings to chicken stock and heat. Now, add egg yolks and cream and cook slowly until thickened a bit. Pour over chicken about ¹/₂ hour before serving. Warm all together. Serve with finely chopped almonds or peanuts, chopped hard-cooked eggs, and finely chopped raw onions. Homemade chutney can also be served.

## Broiled chicken

| | |
|---|---|
| Chicken parts (for 4) | 1 garlic clove |
| 1 T oil | Pinch rosemary and chervil |
| Paprika | Salt and pepper to taste |

Remove skin, if desired. Rub each piece thoroughly with the oil and garlic put through a press, or with garlic powder. Sprinkle both sides with chervil and rosemary (a little goes a long way!), and finally, with some paprika; broil, turning after about 15 minutes. Let cook about 10 minutes longer.

## Baked chicken

| | |
|---|---|
| 1 3-lb frying chicken, cut into pieces | 1 cup light cream, sour cream, or coconut milk or yoghurt |
| 2-3 T oil | Pinch of rosemary |
| ¹/₂ cup fresh mushrooms | Salt and pepper to taste |

Heat oven to moderate. Brown chicken pieces quickly in oil. Place chicken in casserole, cover with cream, mushrooms, and seasonings. Bake about 45 minutes.

## Chicken chow mein (for left-over chicken)

| | |
|---|---|
| 1 T oil | 1/2 cup diced fresh pineapple |
| 1 or more cups diced cooked | (optional) |
| chicken | 1/2 lb fresh sliced mushrooms |
| 1 chopped onion | 1 T soy sauce |
| 3 stalks celery, chopped | |

Brown onions and celery until tender in oil. Add finely sliced mushrooms, soy sauce. Cook a few minutes. Add pineapple and chicken and heat. Serve with whole tomatoes stuffed with cottage cheese.

## Malay chicken

| | |
|---|---|
| 4 or 5 chicken pieces | 2 cloves (optional) |
| 2 garlic cloves, chopped | 1 cup milk mixed with |
| 2 thin slices fresh ginger | 2 egg yolks |
| (or 1/4 t dried) | 2 T chopped onion |
| 4 T oil | 3 T curry powder |
| 1-inch piece cinnamon | 1 large potato |
| (or 1/4 t dried) | |

Gently fry ginger, onion, garlic, cloves, and cinnamon in oil. Make a smooth paste of curry by adding a little water and add to spices in pan, and cook one or two minutes. Peel potato and cut into eighths. Add chicken pieces and potato to spices. Stir well. Add half of the milk and egg combination; then salt and pepper to taste. Heat. Then add rest of milk and simmer all until chicken and potatoes are tender.

## Organ meats

People suffering from gout should avoid organ meats because they contain substances that increase the amount of uric acid in your body.

### Liver

| | |
|---|---|
| 1 lb liver, put through meat chopper | 2 medium onions, chopped fine |
| $^1/_2$ cup ground almonds, raw peanuts or sunflower seed meal | 1 garlic clove, minced |
| $^1/_4$ t ground nutmeg | 2 T cold-pressed oil |
| | Salt and pepper to taste |

Heat oil in skillet. Mix all ingredients. Place by large spoonfuls in oil and brown quickly. Serve immediately. Garnish with sprigs of parsley.

### Liver Chinese-style

| | |
|---|---|
| 1 lb liver, slightly frozen; then cut on diagonal into thin slices | 1 T finely chopped green onion |
| | 1$^1/_2$ T cold-pressed peanut oil |
| 1 cucumber, finely chopped | 2 T soy sauce |
| | 1 t honey |

Mix soy sauce and honey together. Add oil. Mix with liver, in bottom of a casserole. Spread with sliced cucumbers and sprinkle green onions on top. Cover and steam or bake in moderate oven for 25 minutes.

### Portuguese tripe

| | |
|---|---|
| 1 lb honeycomb tripe | 1 garlic clove, minced |
| 2$^1/_2$ cups water | Salt and pepper to taste |
| 1 cup sliced onions | 3 ripe tomatoes |
| $^1/_2$ cup parsley, minced | |

Wash tripe. Simmer in water and a little salt for a couple of hours. Remove tripe and slice into narrow strips. Add other ingredients and simmer about $^1/_2$ hour. Serve hot.

## Stewed heart (Lamb or Beef)

| | |
|---|---|
| 1 heart | 1 T oil |
| $^1/_2$ cup stock or water | Salt and pepper to taste |

Remove veins, arteries, etc., and wash in cold water. Brown in hot oil. Place in small pan, and cover with stock and season. Bake at 150°C, Gas mark 2, 300°F for a couple of hours, turning once. Correct seasonings and serve.

## Kidney casserole

| | |
|---|---|
| 2 t vinegar | $^1/_4$ cup finely diced celery |
| 1 beef kidney or 2 veal or pork kidneys | $^1/_2$ cup fresh mushrooms, quartered |
| 1 small onion chopped, or 3 whole green onions | 2 fresh tomatoes |
| | Salt and pepper to taste |
| $^1/_2$ cup finely diced carrots | Dash of basil and thyme |

Slice kidneys in half, removing all white tissue. Cut into cubes and mix with vinegar. Sear kidneys in a little oil quickly. Remove. Place rest of oil in pan and sauté vegetables. Add kidneys and sauté for about $^1/_4$ hour, turning frequently.

## Sweetbreads

| | |
|---|---|
| 1 lb sweetbreads | 1 onion, finely sliced |
| 2 egg yolks, well beaten, with 1 T milk | 2 sprigs parsely, chopped |
| $^3/_4$ lb mushrooms | 4 T butter |

Remove all membranes of sweetbreads under running water, then dry and dice them. Simmer, covered in a little water about 10 minutes. Melt butter and add sweetbreads, parsley, onion, and water from cooking the sweetbreads. Let it simmer with the sliced mushrooms. Several minutes before serving, add the egg yolk and herbs and salt and pepper to taste. Stir constantly until thickened, and serve immediately.

## Sautéed brains

| | |
|---|---|
| 1 lb veal, pork, lamb, or beef brains | 1/2 tomato |
| 1 egg beaten with 2 T milk | 1 T soy sauce |
| | 2 T butter or oil |

Remove all membranes under running water, dry, and cut into serving pieces. Cover with water and simmer 1/2 hour. Sauté gently until golden brown on both sides. Add other ingredients while stirring and cook for a very short time longer. Serve at once.

## Chicken liver pâté

| | |
|---|---|
| 1 lb chicken livers | 1/4 t ground ginger |
| 3 T oil or butter | 1/4 t allspice |
| 1 medium onion, chopped | Salt and freshly ground pepper |
| 1 bay leaf | to taste |

Melt butter and add onion and seasonings. Stir for a couple of minutes. Add livers, cook gently until golden brown. Remove bay leaf and cool mixture. Blend until smooth in blender or food grinder. Chill. Garnish with paprika or parsley.

## Veal kidneys

| | |
|---|---|
| 3 kidneys, cleaned as above | 2 T cider vinegar |
| 1 T oil | 1 sprig chopped parsley |
| 1/2 chopped onion | Salt and pepper to taste |
| 1 T chopped beef marrow | |

Season the kidneys and brown to golden in oil. Remove kidneys. Cook onion until transparent. Add marrow (made by covering marrow bones with water and cooking about 10 minutes. Then marrow can be pushed out and cut into pieces). Return kidneys to pan and simmer a few minutes. Sprinkle with parsley.

### Loaf of heart

| | |
|---|---|
| 1 lb heart | $^3/_4$ cup of milk |
| 6 green onions or shallots | 1 egg |
| 1 garlic clove | Pinch of thyme and marjoram |
| 3 carrots | |

Wash and drain heart. Cut off tough outer membranes. Put first 4 ingredients through meat grinder. Mix thoroughly, and add the rest of the ingredients. Bake in lightly oiled loaf pan in moderate oven for $^1/_2$ hour.

## Salads (first week)

### Cucumber outriggers*

For individual serving:
Slice one cucumber lengthwise in half. Then cut 1 half in half again, and one piece across. Hollow out the full half and fill with chopped celery, chives, parsley. Season with fresh herbs. Arrange on bed of lettuce. Place sliced cucumber so it resembles an outrigger canoe. Garnish with paprika. Serve with favourite dressing.

### Hi-protein salad*

| | |
|---|---|
| 1 head of lettuce | $^1/_2$ cup sprouts |
| 1 ripe small avocado, sliced | $^1/_4$ cup cheese, crumbled |
| 1 stalk of celery, sliced | 1 hard-boiled egg, crumbled |
| 1 ripe tomato, cut in eighths | Salt or kelp |
| 2 T green onion | Freshly ground pepper |
| Shredded meat, fish, chicken (optional) | |

Prepare lettuce ahead of time; wash and tear into small pieces, wrap in clean towel and refrigerate until ready to serve. Mix all ingredients saving tomatoes, egg, cheese, and meat for last. Pour favourite dressing over all and toss thoroughly.

## Cucumber à la cecil*

| | |
|---|---|
| 2 large cucumbers | Cider vinegar |
| 1 large onion | Salt |
| 1$^1/_2$ T sugar | |

Finely slice the cucumbers and onion. Season with a little salt and 2$^1/_2$ T sugar or honey; place in large bowl and cover with 1 part cider vinegar and 2 parts water. Add $^1/_2$ t oil and a sprinkle of caraway seed. Let stand in refrigerator for several hours before serving.

## Tomato surprise*

| | |
|---|---|
| Ripe tomatoes (1 per serving) | Ground pecan or sprouted |
| Homemade mayonnaise, 1 T | sunflower seeds, $^1/_2$ cup |
| 2 sprigs parsley, minced | |

Cut off top of tomato and scoop out insides. Place pulp in a bowl. Reserve juice for blended vegetable drinks or soups. Mix mayonnaise, parsley, and seeds or nuts with pulp. Sprinkle paprika on top, add a sprig of parsley and place on a bed of lettuce. Chill and serve.

## Spring salad*

| | |
|---|---|
| $^1/_2$ cup shelled June peas | 1 head lettuce, washed and torn |
| $^1/_2$ cup sliced green onion | into bite-sized pieces |
| 1 carrot, grated | 4 radishes, sliced |
| | Several sprigs of mint |

Rub large wooden bowl with garlic clove, discard. Mix your favourite oil and vinegar dressing right in the bowl. Add other ingredients, toss about 20 times and serve immediately.

## Vegetable entrées

### Soybeans

| | |
|---|---|
| 2 cups dried soybeans | 2 cloves garlic, mince |
| 2 cups homemade broth or water | 2 T blackstrap molasses |
| left from cooked vegetables | 1 large onion, sliced |
| 1½ t salt or kelp | 3 T chopped parsley |

Soak soybeans 24 hours in 3 cups of cold water. Change water twice. Simmer between 3 and 4 hours in 2 cups of hot broth. Add more stock if necessary. About ¼ hour before done, add other ingredients. Let water evaporate. Then garnish and serve.

### Carrot apple aspic*

| | |
|---|---|
| 1½ cups diced apples | 1½ T Agar-Agar gelatin |
| 2 cups carrots, grated or diced | Pinch of nutmeg |
| 1 cup apple juice | |

Dissolve gelatin in ½ cup hot water. Stir thoroughly. Add all other ingredients. Chill. Serve on bed of sunflower-seed sprouts.

### Chinese broccoli

| | |
|---|---|
| 1 bunch broccoli | 2 T cold-pressed salad oil |
| 1 t honey | 1 T soy sauce (from health-food |
| 3 cups hot water | store) |

Finely slice broccoli stems on the diagonal into pieces about 1½ by ¼-inch thick. Dissolve honey in hot water. Add broccoli stems first, then flowers broken up into small pieces. Stir gently for one minute. Pour off hot water. Let cool for about 10 minutes. Heat oil in a large skillet. Add broccoli, keep turning the pieces until slightly browned. Add soy sauce and serve immediately.

## Meatless loaf

| | |
|---|---|
| 1 cup grated carrots | 1 clove garlic, crushed |
| 1 cup grated celery | 3 T cold-pressed oil |
| $3/4$ cup peppers, finely minced | 1 cup sprouted seeds or nuts |
| 1 cucumber, minced | Paprika, chives |
| 2 tomatoes, finely chopped | $1/2$ cup thyme |

Mould into loaf. Garnish with parsley, top with paprika and chives. Can be served with homemade gravy.

## Baked vegetables Italian

| | |
|---|---|
| 2 onions, chopped | 1 garlic clove |
| 1 aubergine, large, peeled and sliced | $1/2$ green pepper, seeded and sliced |
| 4 cups tomatoes, chopped into quarters | $1/2$ t basil |
| 1 cup grated natural cheese | $1/2$ t kelp or salt |
| | Freshly ground pepper to taste |
| | 1 cup olive oil |

In skillet, heat about 3 T oil, add garlic; when browned, remove garlic. Brown onions, add tomatoes, seasonings. Simmer $1/2$ hour. Place in casserole, add aubergine and remaining oil, and sprinkle with grated cheese. Bake 30-40 minutes in moderate oven.

## Fresh fruit desserts

### Sandwich isle pudding*

1 cup apricots, dried, soaked (not cooked) in hot water overnight.
2 ripe bananas
1 T honey

Blend all ingredients in a blender to smooth. Place in sherbet glasses and dust with cinnamon or nutmeg.

### Indian apple pudding

6 apples, sliced
$^3/_4$ cup chopped almonds
1$^1/_2$ cups apple juice
1$^1/_2$ T honey

$^1/_4$ cup cream
$^1/_2$ cup raisins (soaked briefly
   to plump)
$^1/_2$ t grated cinnamon

Peel and core apples. Slice into baking dish. Pour cream over apples and dust with cinnamon. Sprinkle nuts on top and bake in 170°C, Gas mark 3, 325°F oven for 15-20 minutes. When cooled serve with cream.

### Pears with raspberry sauce*

1 box fresh raspberries
2 large ripe pears

1 T honey
$^1/_2$ cup blanched, slivered
   almonds

Peel and halve pears. Blend or purée raspberries with honey. Pour over pears. Sprinkle with almonds.

### Fresh apple sauce*

2 cups apples
1 T or more honey

Pinch cinnamon
$^1/_2$ cup sundried raisins

Core and quarter the apples, leaving skins on. Blend apples with water or apple juice until all is smooth. Add the seasonings and the raisins. Blend about 30 seconds more. Serve or chill in refrigerator.

## Banana cream pie*

| | |
|---|---|
| 2 cups crushed nuts | *Filling* |
| 3/4 cup butter | 3 very ripe bananas |
| 1 T honey | 1 cup of whipped cream |
| | 1/2 t vanilla |
| | Pinch of nutmeg |

For crust: Melt butter and press crushed nuts, butter and sweetening into pie pan with fingers. Sprinkle a tablespoon of cold water on top and press firmly so mixture will adhere to side and bottom of pan. Filling is prepared by mashing bananas and folding in whipped cream and vanilla. Sprinkle with a pinch of powdered nutmeg. Chill in refrigerator until serving time.

### For your action

- Every time you step into your kitchen, be aware of the effect of water and heat on the nutritive value of food. Devise ways of cooking your favourite foods as little as possible – as little heat, as little water. Save cooking water for later use instead of pouring it down the drain.
- Use juicers or blenders more in food preparation. Try some of the recipes in this chapter. Let them trigger your own ingenuity in cooking less, enjoying more.
- Remember also, and this is vitally important for more rapid recovery from arthritis, the simpler your menus the quicker you get better. For the fastest recovery have only one meal a day and let it be some lightly sautéed seafood, a raw mixed vegetable or fruit salad, and raw milk. Alternate the seafood with beef liver, or lamb kidneys, lamb hearts, or pork liver.
- You will be amazed at the health you will enjoy – especially in diminishing arthritic pains.

# CHAPTER 9

# Keys to Rapid Joint Repair
# of Arthritic Damage

The title of this chapter means what it says. Despite all you may have been told, bones and joints are not always *permanently* damaged even when ravished by a decade or more of crippling arthritis and even when you are in the so-called golden years. Nature wants you to function perfectly. Here in this chapter is how you can help her.

The home cure for arthritis in this book is quite simple, as you have discovered in the preceding chapters. Following is a summary of The book's progress to this point:

- A day of fast to rest the organs.
- A week, or more if needed, of only raw fresh fruits, raw fresh vegetables, and liver.
- A continuing diet of the right foods, avoiding processed and other harmful foods.
- Continuous attention from start of treatment to the organs of elimination, especially the *bowels*!
- A programme of increasing motion to encourage better blood circulation and regeneration of tissues.

These are steps that can all be taken right in your own home. In most cases, these are the only steps that need to be taken to bring about a permanent cure.

"But what about me? I've had arthritis for eight years. I'm now 70 years old. I have no more pain. The heat and swelling are gone. But will I ever be able to walk erect again?"

What this person is really asking is: Can bones and joints be restored?

The answer is "YES."

Nevertheless, even if you were totally conscientious in observing the five requisites to cure listed above, there would still be one major obstacle standing in your way.

## A major obstacle and what to do about it

"There is nothing medical science can do to cure you, Mrs Smith. You might just as well decide right now that you will have to adjust as best you can to the effects of arthritis."

The doctor's voice is comforting and he is the typical M.D. It is the voice of authority. There is no recourse to a higher authority. "Arthritis cannot be cured. Arthritis cannot be cured." How many times have you heard this? May I shift the scene to another location. It may seem unrelated. But there is a real connection and an important one.

It is a room in a cheap hotel. The body of a young woman is sprawled on the floor. A suicide note is pinned on the bed. An empty glass is lying near her right hand. The police check the bathroom. There are two bottles standing side by side – mouthwash and deadly carbolic acid. Routinely they check the glass. It contains only traces of mouthwash.

The woman had mistakenly drunk relatively harmless mouthwash instead of death-dealing carbolic acid. But she died anyway.

Such can be the power of suggestion.

Most doctors use this power of suggestion constructively. They are optimistic and hopeful. They may feel uncertainty but they express confidence. This is good.

### The placebo

They also make frequent use of the placebo.

Here is what it is and how it works.

You tell the doctor your symptoms. He examines you. He can find nothing really wrong. But he does not tell you this. Instead, he shakes his head knowingly and writes out a prescription. "One tablet every two hours. Call me in a few days." You take the prescription to the white-coated pharmacist. He tells you to come back in a few minutes (it must be a complicated mixture of drugs, you think). You return, it is ready. You take the prescribed doses. The symptoms disappear.

The complicated mixture usually is sugar.

Yes, those little white sugar pills, endowed with the power of suggestion, have cured you.

## The power of suggestion

The power of suggestion works via the subconscious. This is the automatic computer that controls the operation of your body and often your emotional reactions, attitudes, and behaviour.

A person with rose fever walks into a room, sees a vase of red roses and begins to sneeze. It does not matter that they are plastic imitations. Of course, if this fact is disclosed, the sneezing stops!

How many billions of colds have been caused by well-meaning mothers who instruct their children, "Don't get your feet wet or you'll catch a cold." Or, "Don't sit in a draught or you'll catch a cold."

Surgeons and their operating-room staff, after a number of cases where casual gloomy remarks have caused setbacks to their patients, now know to refrain from such talk. Even in a state of anaesthesia, the subconscious mind records what it hears and programmes the patient accordingly.

I must say the Arthritis Foundation tries to be optimistic and to give readers of its pamphlets positive suggestions. But it still comes out sounding pretty dim.

For example: No case is hopeless.

Or: Is there any cure for rheumatoid arthritis? – No, but serious crippling can be avoided in almost all instances.

In his book, *Arthritis, Medicine and the Spiritual Laws,** Loring T. Swaim, M.D., recognizes the effect of the mind on the body. His book was recommended by doctors and clergy alike. It helped the reader maintain a positive attitude.

I want more than that from you.

* Chilton Book Company, Philadelphia, 1962.

- I want you to *know* that you can be cured.
- I want you to *know* that joints and bones in arthritis patients on the arthritis-cure programme are being restored every day
- I want you to *know* that your joints and your bones, if you are on the arthritis-cure programme, are being restored today.
- If you don't know this implicitly and without one single, even ephemeral, shadow of a doubt, then stop reading right here and now and look very carefully at the before and after X-ray pictures on page 173.

Yes, nature renews tissues, heals wounds, repairs, organs. And nature restores bones and joints if you let her.

### How we can get in our own way or out of it

They say that childbirth is a lot easier for women in rural areas and undeveloped countries where it is understood to be just one more of our natural functions. There is less tension, less pain.

In the civilized world, however, young girls are constantly subjected to tales of horror of childbirth. When the event approaches for one of them, she is naturally ready for the worst. She is tense, expects excruciating pain from the pressure. She tightens up. She gets what she expects.

You, too, have been brainwashed. You have heard and seen endless cases where arthritics have gone from one doctor to another, tried one treatment after another, one gadget after another, only to have their hopes dashed down.

They have told you of the futility.

They have permitted you to share their despair.

**The case of Mrs A. B.'s husband**

Please suffer this real-life drama along with Mrs A. B. I'll make it worth your while. She writes about her husband Bob:

"It really started, I think, way back in 1947 or '48. Bob was troubled then with pains in the lower back. The doctor diagnosed it as trouble with the sacroiliac. He rested for a while and then went back to work at his job as a carpenter.

"Some time later, when he started having trouble again, a back brace, similar to a stiffly boned corset, was recommended. He wore this for quite a long time. Later, he would wear it for a day or two whenever the back seemed to be acting up. Then for several years everything seemed all right.

"Perhaps, it really wasn't. Perhaps, he became used to the pain and learned to live with it. Or perhaps, I was just too busy with three children to notice whether he was in pain or not. While he grunted occasionally when he stood up or got out of bed, he didn't complain of anything. Once he asked for a mustard plaster.

"One weekend when we had a three-day holiday, we had sealed off a closet door in one of the bedrooms prior to going ahead with a plan to break through a wall and enlarge our living room. Bob was bent over picking up some old plaster – he stood up and said, "Call and make an appointment with Dr P."

"He saw Dr P. who sent him to a diagnostician, who sent him to an internist. Test after test was done to locate the cause of the pain in the lower back. No one could put his finger on what was causing it. All tests showed everything in good working order. He seemed to be in less pain – possibly because he, at least, knew that everything that had been checked was okay.

"Weeks later he was again feeling miserable. He would be sitting in a chair talking and suddenly would wince and his legs would pull up towards his chest.

"He complained of pains in his chest and my first thought was his heart. But then I had another theory: He had broken an ankle when in service and walked on it before it had attention. Because of that, one leg was a little shorter than the other. Perhaps, I said, this was the cause of the backache and just a little correction in his shoe would put the spine back in its proper place. He was ready to try anything. He went to Dr C., an orthopaedist, who X-rayed him extensively. The next day Dr C. called. It was Marie Strümpell's arthritis.

"Radiation treatment was given at a hospital. The treatment wasn't bad, but the after-effects were miserable. Bob would come home, have dinner, and in about an hour start upchucking it for several hours. A year later more X-rays were taken. They showed the problem to have been arrested but still concentrated in the spot.

"Now, several years went by. There were good times and bad. He learned to live with the pain, take aspirin, or soak in a hot tub. Many nights, I would wake to the sound of water running in the bathroom at three or four a.m.

"He had been an easy-going person. When we first moved here the boys in the neighbourhood used to call for him to come out and have a baseball 'catch.' He helped them build a club house, took them sleigh riding at the park. He was fun to be with, always ready to help neighbours with a project or a problem. The change was probably gradual. But suddenly to me he was impossible. It became more difficult to please him. I would hope he would go to bed early so that the kids and I could breathe more freely. There were times when I thought of consulting a psychiatrist.

"After many miserable months, I talked him into going to see Dr Campbell ..."

I interrupt the letter here to remind you that I was faced at this point with a man who was conditioned to expect failure. He was told again and again that there was no cure. He was repeatedly told that at best he could only be made more comfortable. Even this was proving to be a hollow promise as his pain continued and became a dreary, heavy way of life.

When I saw him for the first time, I could feel this hopelessness. Although he did not say much, I could sense that he was holding back. "Whatever you have in store for me, Doctor, it won't work."

I fought this first. I gave it top priority. I told him of other cases we had treated and the cures that had taken place or were taking place. I showed him X-rays. I brought it closer to home for him by relating the 'miraculous' progress of his wife's friend who recommended me to her. I could not tell whether I was getting through to him but I went on anyway with his first-week's instructions and he left.

Now let's see what happened when he got home. His wife's letter continues:

**Mrs A. B.'s story continued**

"When he came home I asked him what the doctor had said. 'He's a nut. It won't work. He's a nut.'

"Dr Campbell had recommended bed rest, but since Bob doesn't get paid unless he works that was impossible. He went on the strict food diet, went to work, came home, showered, went to bed, had dinner and went to sleep. Because all the foods were things he didn't like and could never eat before, I ate exactly what he had. He cooperated. His first visit was on a Tuesday and he was to return the next Monday. I remember a neighbour asking me that Monday morning if I thought Bob would keep the appointment and if he felt any better. I replied that I didn't know whether he felt any better (there hadn't been much conversation other than 'ugh' when he saw his dinner) but that I knew I did.

"Well, he went that night. He came home from the visit. No remarks this time. He stuck to the diet and in a month was the old Bob everyone liked so well."

*Expectation and belief*

Expectation and belief are important. More than that, they are essential.

First, they motivate you to follow the cure procedures.

Second, they create the mental climate conducive to change.

Bob was playing it safe with the "he's a nut" expression. He was preparing to save face in case of failure with "I told you so."

The X-rays, the cure of his wife's friend, and other successes were too powerful to be ignored. They got a foothold on his subconscious mind. They were enough to motivate him to eat foods he would not otherwise have put up with. They were enough to make him look for, even expect, changes. Those changes were evident in two or three days. He was reticent to announce them as there had been remissions like this before.

Even at his second visit, I sensed his reservations, though also an increased attention and receptivity to direction.

The rest was easy.

I cite this case because it turned on such a hair. It could have gone the other way. I might never have seen him. Or, I might never have motivated him. Finally, through a credibility gap, he could have slowed his cure and perpetuated arthritis symptoms through the faithful servomechanism of his subconscious mind. In other words, he could have stood in his own way.

The greatest credibility gap seems to exist among older people. They are likely to accept arthritis as a condition of age. They are more likely to have had arthritis for a longer period, and grown accustomed to it. They are less likely to accept the possibility of bone improvement at their age.

Arthritis can be cured at any age – with cooperation and expectation.

Cooperation and expectation keep us from standing in our own way.

## How to put your mind to work for you

Some people not only get out of their own way, they actually harness the creative faculty of the mind to help nature along.

Of course, I'm referring to the power of thinking positively which has been proven effective in every line of human endeavour including health.

If we imagine and fear ailments, it acts as a depressant to health. If we visualize ourselves in radiant good health, it moves us quite perceptibly in that direction.

If a doctor is not aware of this – and most doctors are very much aware of it – he is inclined to take patients at their face value.

For instance, woman A comes in complaining how bad her arthritis pains have been despite treatment. Woman B comes in radiating optimism and ignoring her pain. Woman A is apparently the sicker person – judging by face value. But she may not be.

Woman B might be sicker but I'll wager she will recover more quickly than woman A, all else being equal. The difference is her positive attitude.

If you are on the mend, do not think of the suffering you still have, think of the improvements you can enjoy tomorrow. Also, think of your bones and joints as returning to normal. Know what a healthy knee or hip should look like. Visualize yourself with healthy bone and joint structure.

The golfer who addresses the ball and dwells on avoiding the rough on one side and the water hazard on the other is risking driving into one or the other. The successful pros concentrate their attention on where they want the ball to go, not where they don't want it to go.

Arthritis sufferers – think positively! Visualize yourself getting progressively healthier. See every arthritis problem disappearing, every bone and joint being restored to the way it should be. Then watch nature respond as you help her as outlined in this book.

## Why bones respond even at advanced age

"No Cure, But Help Is Found for Arthritis." So reads a recent headline. Additional 'evidence' reinforces a hard-core belief about arthritis.

This particular story appeared recently in the *Honolulu Star Bulletin* following a medical association meeting. The Texas physician-biochemist who reported on arthritis noted that two surgical procedures offered hope:

1  The excision (cutting out) of inflamed tissue.
2  The total joint replacement by gluing in a metal substitute.

He also reported there was hope in the development of immuno-suppressive drugs.

*Not one word about the cause!*

Take a look at the two examples of bone improvement in Plates I and II. Plate I shows the condition of a patient with a well-advanced case of the supposedly incurable disease, Paget's, of the shinbone (the 'before' picture). The 'after' picture, Plate II, shows unmistakable improvement of the condition six months later.

I am not going to tell you how old my patient was in this case.

Some of you may be older and be inclined to say, "Well, it cannot happen at my age, I'd have to be younger." Don't fool yourself. It can happen at any age!

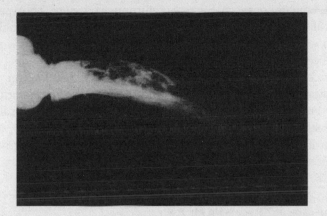

PLATE I. Before: Dark portions or spots on this X-ray show softening of the bone in an advanced case of Paget's disease of the shinbone, deemed incurable.

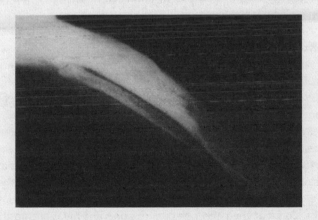

PLATE II. After: Note the replacement of calcium and phosphorus six months later shown by the light areas. The bone is now stronger and no longer flexible.

Nature abhors an abnormal condition. Take away the cause of that condition healthfully and nature will seek to restore it to normal condition.

Remember this: New cells are being formed in your body by the millions every day. Soft tissues are renewed much faster than hard bone, but bones are at least partially renewed every few years, even at the slower replacement rate of the octogenarian or older.

Bones move towards normal while you sleep, while you work, while you play if you follow the guidance in this book.

Once the cause is removed – the ingestion of chemicals and of denatured and processed foods – and the building blocks for the body are provided – fresh, raw, nutritious foods – new healthy bone cells begin to replace faulty bone cells.

Given improper nutrition, count on cell imperfection. Given proper nutrition, count on cell perfection.

### The case of 72-year-old Mr J. K.

Can you imagine raw fruits and raw vegetables reinforced with the other ingredients on the arthritis-cure diet changing a condition in a cervical spine in just a week or two? Let Mr J. K. tell you: He was 72 years old when I met him.

"I'm very happy to be among the living, so I can report what took place.

"Four years ago, I started to get pains in my arms and fingers. First, it only occurred mid-day and in only one hand, just fleeting stabs. Gradually, it progressed, became more severe, steadier, went over to the left shoulder and hand.

"By this time, I went to see a physician who gave me aspirin which alleviated the pain somewhat in the beginning. As time went on, 12 aspirins a day didn't make any impression. I sought another doctor who pronounced it brachial neuritis and gave me some other drug called 'Indocin.' Then we tried 'Sterazolidin.' These drugs had a slight numbing effect on both the pain and my head, mostly my head. I began to get nauseated, so had to reduce the amount and finally had to quit them.

"Other medications were tried with no effect. Finally, I was put in a hospital in Brooklyn, where I stayed six weeks. The condition was diagnosed as angina pectoris.

"When I left the hospital, the condition was somewhat worse. I decided to go to Miami, Florida and enter a hospital there. I stayed in that hospital for three weeks and was examined by orthopaedic specialists who discovered I had arthritis of the cervical spine. They told me that nothing could be done and I'd just have to live with it.

"The condition became intolerable. In fact, there were several occasions while walking along the street, when I would suddenly lose consciousness and wake up in some hospital, being treated for a heart attack. By this time, the disc spaces in my cervical spine had degenerated to a point where they were practically non-existent. The bodies of the vertebrae had overgrown with bone where, in certain positions, they would completely pinch off my spinal cord and cause me to lose consciousness.

"Of course, I could not work for a long time, never knowing when I would lose consciousness. Nor could I sleep, due to pains constantly in my shoulders and arms.

"All these symptoms were completely cleared up in a very short time, after I started getting treatments from Dr Campbell. As I recall now, I do not believe I had any loss of consciousness after the first week of treatment. It was fantastic! Within three weeks, the pain had left my shoulders, arms, and hands.

"Naturally, I was placed on a nutritional programme that was very odd to me at the time, but I was willing to try anything and have stuck with it ever since.

"The treatment deserves world-wide recognition. No human being should have to go through the living hell I did."

Mr J. K. was back to work in two months.

Bone improvement takes place in your own home. It took place in Mr J. K.'s.

## The true-proven cure for arthritis

There is not now, and I doubt if there ever will be a pill for curing arthritis. The only cure I know of is the cure in this book. It is working faithfully for those who apply it faithfully. It will work for you. But no drug company will promote it because they will not profit from it. Since no profit is involved, no money is available to spread the word.

Since it is a cure based largely on diet, doctors are loath to use it. They have enough problems with obesity patients, diabetics, and others. Trying to encourage anybody to stay on a strict diet is a thankless task for a doctor. He would much rather hold the reins himself than hand them over to the patient who may or may not steer the proper diet course.

These may all seem like reasons to permit patients to continue to suffer year in and year out. But there is much more behind the scenes.

There are respected nutritionists, some with large universities, who receive large consultant fees from food processors and who are inclined to pooh-pooh, as they have in the past, any diet that eliminated their processor-client products. The number of empty calories and arthritis-laden calories that have been peddled in the name of 'fortified,' 'refined,' 'enriched', and 'balanced' is scandalous to me.

Behind the scenes, too, is a reticence to be called wrong. Many professional people persevere along an increasingly doubtful path rather than admit that past efforts were not on the right track. It is not a characteristic exclusive to medical men. It is human.

Not behind the scenes, but ever evident as part of the modem scene, is the continuing campaign on behalf of processed foods by their makers, together with their continuing campaign of 'quackery' accusations against those who advocate natural, organic foods.

I wonder how many of them have arthritis?

## Take the load off rejuvenating bones and joints

Earlier in this chapter I gave you some mental ways you can help nature restore your affected bones and joints. There are physical ways, too.

First of all, follow the instructions for rest and movement in chapter 6. Take the load off an especially overworked area such as the knees or back.

You may be told that it is the strain of this work that has caused wear and tear on the bones or joints. This is not true. *The cause is the weakening of the bones and joints due to wrong diet*. Then the arthritis appears at the point where this weakness proves your undoing – the knees for one type of work, the hands for another, the back for a third.

Assuming you are abstaining from the wrong foods, eating the right foods, encouraging efficient elimination, and improving circulation with motion, you can consider the use of some mechanical aids to take the load off your healing bones and joints as they heal.

Osteoarthritis of the lower back often involves pressure on nerves. This can be quite painful even after the cure has started. Aspirin and hot baths help but those sharp twinges may still persist. Osteopathic manipulation of the area involved will be very effective and in some cases is a must.

If the knees are involved, the elastic strapping used by athletes is supportive. Where the top of the back or the neck and arms are affected, there are home-traction devices that are not too expensive which can be used to relieve this pinching of the nerves. Yet, here too osteopathy provides the best relief by removing the congestion and thus allowing a good blood flow to get to the diseased area.

The drawback of mechanical traction with home devices or in hospital, is that they can't feel when the body has had enough. At a certain point the muscles 'fight back' with more contraction to prevent overstretching. Only a skilled pair of hands can feel when the traction has gone far enough.

Nature's healing powers make their best progress when we sleep or just rest. The body uses less energy, fuel, and nutrients for work and activity, also less energy for digestion and other maintenance activities, and is able to devote more energy and nutrients to repair and rehabilitation.

It stands to reason that, after the diet and elimination cure is underway, a housewife with arthritis in her knees is not giving them a proper chance to repair themselves if she repeatedly kneels down to scrub. And the same applies to the bus driver who may have the problem in his elbows, or the plumber or mechanic with hip or back problems who must constantly contort himself to get into tight spots.

The choice might be enforced idleness for a much longer period. The temporary restraint is a small price to pay for full recovery.

## Two cases of proven bone restoration

Arthritis cures do take place. *Age is no barrier.* Legs strengthen. Hips recover. Knees return to normal. Fingers improve. Backs straighten. My files are full of case histories that read like miracles.

A 60-year-old housewife suffered from generalized rheumatoid arthritis that involved her ankles, knees, shoulders, elbows, wrists, and hands. The disease had been in progress for one year before I first saw her. During that period the disease became steadily worse despite medical care at a New York hospital where cortisone was prescribed. The last doctor she saw was an arthritis specialist. He informed her that it was inevitable that she be permanently confined to a wheel chair.

She became almost totally incapacitated. She was unable to dress herself. She could feed herself only with great difficulty.

On her first visit to me she was able to navigate without the aid of crutches or cane but had to be assisted by her husband in order to walk. To climb stairs was extremely difficult. She was immediately placed on the nutritional programme outlined in this book. The cortisone was discontinued immediately.

Remember, all affected joints were swollen, hot, and painful. Her skin had that typical clammy, sandy feeling.

When the diet was initiated, osteopathic treatments were given as well as the other treatment adjuncts described in previous chapters.

Within one week the swelling had greatly diminished, the pain had left, except for extreme movements, and aspirin, which had been taken at the rate of 12 per day, was reduced to three per day. At the end of a month she was able to assist her husband in his business which she hadn't been able to do for over two years.

At the end of the second month she was walking jauntily along Fifth Avenue in New York City, when she met the arthritis specialist who had told her she would eventually end up in a wheel chair. He was amazed at her present condition and inquired what she had done. She told him she was on a diet and was getting osteopathic treatments. He asked her if she would mind telling him what the diet was; since it had done so much for her, perhaps it would do the same for some of his patients. She told him the major points but referred him to me for the details. I never heard from him.

She went on to complete recovery. She uses no medication, has no pain, nor any evidence that she ever had arthritis.

A 66-year-old housewife with no children had arthritis of all joints of the upper and lower extremities for 25 years. The ankles and wrists were markedly deformed. The elbows could be moved but not extended. Many doctors had treated her over the years. Visits to four different spas throughout the world were of no avail.

In this case constipation was present. It was a critical factor and very difficult to overcome. This delayed recovery.

Two months went by before the pain left all the joints. Even then there was some residual pain in the wrists. Heat still persisted in these joints until two and a half months later. Then the pain left and the elbows could be fully extended. This was something she had not been able to do for 15 years.

Prednisone 5 mg was administered in this case for two months at the rate of one tablet three times a day, together with the other treatments both at home and in the office which I have detailed for you.

She has completely recovered, and has moved to Florida.

## What happens in severe arthritis afflictions

Some cases are not so dramatic. People suffering from Marie Strümpell's disease, otherwise known as spondylitis or spinal arthritis, must act within the first five years from its beginning or it will be too late.

Here's what happens.

The spine segments proliferate. In a few years the whole spine can become one solid bone, fixed, rigid, bent forward. You have probably seen its victims walking, quite bent over, head held somewhat like a turtle's to avoid staring constantly at the ground.

Under orthodox treatment, these patients never get well. Under our treatment, the pain stops and repair starts. If it has progressed for five years or more, however, motion may not be re-established at the sites of bony ankylosis. Still, to stop the pain and halt the progress of this disease is a dramatic happening for any sufferer.

To me the case histories of cures follow the same definite pattern of progress. For example, a 75-year-old man suffers the pain of acute rheumatoid arthritis in all joints. He is bedridden. In one week the pain is gone. In two weeks he is on his feet. In three weeks his deformed fingers straighten enough to hold the steering wheel and drive the car.

It happens to him.

It happens to her.

It can happen to you – whatever your age.

## For your action

- Put your mind to work alongside of nature by wiping the mental slate clean of all negative conditioning about the body's ability to restore bones damaged by arthritis.
- Instead, visualize your bones and joints as they once were and how they can once again be.
- Help nature physically, too, by not subjecting rejuvenating joints and bones to undue work and stress loads even though the pain is gone.

# CHAPTER 10

# Medications and Treatments – Those That May Help and Those That May Hinder

Health care has become dominated by inoculations, serums, pills, capsules, and medications of all types. Yet arthritis remains untouched by these powerful medical agents. "We cannot cure arthritis because we don't know what it is," remains medical science's standard statement. This chapter helps you to understand the latest medical approaches to arthritis and to steer your own best course for your arthritis cure.

You, the arthritis sufferer, have been the more or less innocent victim of body pollution.

It has occurred in your own home.

It can be cured in your own home.

No warning bells, sirens, or gongs were sounded when you sat down each morning to a breakfast of refined sugar and flour products or a dinner of other 'civilized' foods.

No triumphal trumpets will blare when you eat natural foods and the heat, pain, and swelling subside and joints return to normal.

For some people, this is hard to take. First, they don't like to accept the blame for their own condition. Second, they prefer to have somebody in there fighting the enemy along with them.

Enter the micro-organism.

## Health wreckers

Whenever the level of plant or animal health goes down, invaders arrive. If the soil does not supply the plant with what it needs, insects move in on the vulnerable leaves and stems.

If nutrition is less than adequate for man or animal, or if the environment supplies tension and anxiety to erode man's health, the germ and the virus have a field day.

Conventional medicine has come to look upon these little creatures as the cause of most diseases rather than as the result of a lowered resistance due to a more basic cause. This mistaken notion is supported by the fact that when the micro-organisms are destroyed the specific symptoms disappear. But if the resistance to disease is not restored you can expect a return of the little health wreckers.

Since arthritis is a state of lowered resistance and obvious malfunctioning of the body, infections often occur along with it. This has given rise to a concept that the arthritis is caused by the infection – but don't you believe it.

## Infections and arthritis

Not too long ago, if a person suffering from arthritis was found to have inflamed tonsils, out came the tonsils in an operation. Yet the arthritis condition went merrily on its way, absolutely untouched by the absence of tonsils.

If a person suffering from arthritis had a tooth or two or three that were subnormal in some way, they were deemed to be the cause of the arthritis and out they came along with a few on each side and above to boot. Yet the arthritis condition went merrily on its way, absolutely unaffected by the absence of the teeth.

Physicians are getting away from that concept – slowly. Recently, a man came to me with rheumatoid arthritis of the fingers of the right hand and of the left knee. His doctor recommended the extraction of his upper wisdom teeth. You can figure out the reasoning yourself. "Arthritis must be caused by an infection. Wisdom teeth are often the site or focus of an infection. Wisdom teeth are not absolutely essential. Nothing to lose, maybe something to gain – out."

Net result: a man suffering from rheumatoid arthritis without his upper wisdom teeth!

Most enlightened physicians today know that these so-called foci of infection do not cause arthritis. They are merely the added signs of a diseased body, a body not equipped to stand the normal rigours of existence.

Infected tonsils, rectal fistulae, infected teeth, are never the cause of arthritis. These are additional symptoms of the body's general deterioration because of the lack of adequate nutrition.

Don't get me wrong. I don't mean to say that we should ignore these infections. They need to be treated too. In fact, if tonsils or a tooth becomes infected to a degree that its recovery is not likely, then it becomes an additional source of pollution for the whole body. At that point, its removal will hasten the cure for arthritis.

*But the infection is not the basic cause of the arthritis.* They both stem from the same cause. They are brothers under the skin – an undernourished skin of an undernourished, poorly evacuated body.

## The real miracle behind some arthritis drugs

Understanding this basic cause for arthritis, we are still faced with some interesting facts.

### The gold treatment

A chemical compound containing gold is prescribed for injections for a person suffering from rheumatoid arthritis. The doctor prescribing this knows it will not cure the arthritis but that occasionally this treatment will reduce the severity of rheumatoid inflammation.

The prescribing doctor does not consider this a miracle drug, but I do.

How a toxic substance which can kill the patient – like a gold compound – actually reduces arthritic inflammation for even a brief period is a mystery.

Perhaps this gold is so much more lethal or deadly in the body than the general deterioration caused by processed foods that it causes the body to marshal its defences in an intense way that *temporarily* relieves the arthritis pains.

The sad part is that the arthritis remains. And once gold has been administered for a length of time, the body may never be able to attain with healthful foods that delicate chemical balance on the plus side that eventually leads to cure.

The golden hope turns to a leaden weight on health prospects for the patient.

There are other drugs that doctors use knowing that they will not cure, but they are satisfied in the knowledge that they are doing the best they can for their patients.

## Cortisone

Cortisone and cortisone-related drugs, called steroids, can have a dramatic effect on the inflammation in rheumatoid arthritis. In a matter of hours a patient may feel much better and become more active.

Here again we have a miracle. For these too, are substances that are not tolerated by the body and are unsafe. As you increase the doses, the greater will be the alleviation of arthritis *symptoms* but the worse will be the side effects of the steroids – with the obvious end result of no net progress secured.

There are other drugs being used now and more being developed – all with that seemingly inevitable combination of hope and threat.

## Various other drugs used for coping with arthritis

Phenylbutazone also reduces inflammation but substitutes its own symptoms.

Antimalarials are a family of drugs under a number of trade names, but all are derivatives of quinine. They promise arthritis relief with one hand and the possibility of anaemia with the other.

Indomethacin is a relative newcomer with the price of its relief – I repeat, relief not cure – still not thoroughly recognized but nevertheless already spotted as 'minor side effects.'

Indomethacin (Indocid, Indolar), is known as a non-steroidal anti-inflammatory drug (NSAID). A wide range of side effects have been reported involving the stomach, liver, blood changes, circulatory system, skin, and eyes.

## The parade of drugs still to come

Many medical doctors are themselves tired of the drug approach. They would like to see a return to the general practitioner's image as a family doctor who emphasizes friendly counselling, proper diet, an occasional trip to get away from it all, and rest.

But then along come some more 'bottled' discoveries that offer an expedient albeit fragmented attack on the problem.

Research has been going on for over five years on the effects of a drug known as cyclophosamide or cytoxin, a type of nitrogen mustard developed in Germany to combat the body's rejection of transplants. Doctors at the Southwestern Clinic and Research Institute in Arizona noticed that the drug affected lymphocytes, a white blood cell, in such a way that arthritis was mysteriously arrested in about 25 per cent of the persons treated and improvements noted in other patients. Side effects included loss of hair, intestinal upsets – so far. The drug must be taken daily to maintain its benefits, but, of course, this frequency maintains and possibly increases side effects.

More elusive are the side effects of a more natural discovery, histidine, an amino acid natural to the body. One to six grains a day cause marked improvements in some patients but no improvements in others, according to tests being run in a Brooklyn hospital. There are probably no side effects; but there are probably no benefits either except where patients are short of this particular nutrient.

## Drugs will not cure arthritis

Let's face it. There are no drugs that will cure arthritis. Nor is it likely that there will ever be any.

It is like hoping for a chemical to pour on the city dump to make it go away. The only way it would go away is if all the waste were removed and no new waste added. And for arthritis sufferers, that's the name of the game – first get rid of your body wastes and toxins as shown in this book.

When cortisone first came out, the manufacturers claimed it to be such a cure. 'This was supported by many authorities and played up as such by a national magazine. It may have been an unintentional deception but it nevertheless had all the ill effects of a cruel hoax.

### How your blood chemistry can be affected by drugs

Just like gold compounds, a long series of cortisone treatments can affect the blood chemistry It becomes irreparably altered and does not then respond to the natural dietary and elimination treatment that would otherwise cure. A person can therefore count himself out of an arthritis cure as provided in this book.

## Some helpful cortisone derivatives

As I mentioned in an earlier chapter; there have now been developed some derivatives of cortisone that are helpful in the cure of arthritis – *providing the diet and elimination regime is also being followed*.

The composition of cortisone, in its original state, contained many chemicals not relating to the principal factor that reduced inflammation. Some of these chemicals were harmful and produced harmful side effects and after effects.

Now the active principals of the drug have been isolated. We have prednisolone, prednisone, and the injectable hydrocortisone acetate. All these are often helpful in obtaining a more rapid recovery from the pain of arthritis.

For example, in those cases with arthritis of the knees where there is a great deal of swelling and extra fluid in the joint, the liquid is withdrawn and 1 cubic centimetre comprising 25 or 50 milligrams hydrocortisone is reinjected. This procedure often slows down the recurrence of extra fluid and in some cases, when the swelling is not too great, even prevents it from returning. At the same time, it alleviates pain in a great many cases. If it is not injected exactly in the joint space, it may increase the pain for a while.

Hydrocortisone is actually only an anti-inflammatory drug and *in no way helps to repair the damage created by arthritis*. Repair can only be brought about by increased healthful blood flow. The blood must carry the necessary nutrients for repair. And you now know how to ensure this.

If, in spite of all your efforts, you still have pain and feel that steroids may be necessary you must discuss this with your doctor or specialist who are the only people able to prescribe them for you. The doctor, being aware of the side effects of steroids, will probably wish to try NSAIDs first.

There is a safer option available – acupuncture. This method of treatment, used increasingly in the most progressive modern medical and naturopathic institutions, originated in China several thousand years ago. Certain combinations of points, when treated by the fine needles or heated by the burning moxa herbs used by acupuncture practitioners, will encourage the body to produce more of its own natural steroid secretions. The treatment is gentle and painless.

## More about aspirin

Aspirin remains the best palliative or reliever of all as it causes the fewest side effects. But, as I have stated before, there *are* side effects even to aspirin. The most common and incipiently dangerous is the pitting of the stomach resulting in internal haemorrhaging.

New aspirins are being developed, usually along the lines of 'buffering,' to soften the impact on the stomach wall. Some-aspirins are being marketed to cut down the massiveness of the dose by releasing the acetylsalicylic acid slowly over a period of 12 hours or more.

I usually prescribe one or two 5-gram aspirin tablets, three or four times a day for a day or two. Then I cut it down to one such tablet three or four times a day. This may have to be maintained for the first week or ten days of the diet cure. After that, it may be temporarily necessary during weather changes but then will come that day when even weather changes will bring no pain.

Palliatives all – merely temporary relief. As curatives, none qualifies.

## The futility of most drug discoveries

Man's effort to conquer nature often seems crowned with success. But then nature seems to have the last say.

Since the time of Pasteur there has been a parade of medical 'triumphs.'Yet, where are we? Let's consider the factual situations.

We are still a disease-ridden people. As fast as one disease is licked, one or two new ones pop up to take its place, or else the remaining old ones become more prevalent.

The miracle drug is used. Then the body becomes allergic or immune to its use. Or the germs that it originally killed become immune to it, or new varieties of the microbe evolve that survive the drug. And if none of these things happens, then there is always the likelihood that in curing one illness the patient can develop an iatrogenic illness – that is, an undesirable and often fatal side effect of a drug.

Little wonder that the unorthodox methods of health care such as those used by herbalism, naturopathy, chiropractic, and osteopathy are gaining in popularity.

Even those who stick with orthodox medicine are no longer accepting those pills blindly but are now asking searching questions about what they are and what they do.

### A woman's experience with arthritis drugs

"In 1957, at age 40, I first noticed that the knuckles of my middle fingers and my left thumb were swollen to the extent that I could not bend those fingers and could not grasp anything with my left hand. Within a couple of months, even though I had gone to a couple of medical doctors, the condition grew worse and I could hardly move my neck, arms, or legs.

"During the next nine years, I went to eight other doctors, taking cortisone, or gold treatments, or pills, but I still had pain and stiffness in my arms and legs, and my right knee was swollen immensely. It was therefore very hard for me to commute to and from the city each day to business as I had great difficulty in walking and ascending or descending stairs.

"On my first visit to Dr Campbell, he drained 200 cc's [cubic centimetres] of fluid from my right knee, used the neuromuscular stimulator, gave me an injection of Hydrocortisone (25 mg), and an osteopathic treatment. He also gave me a diet to follow.

"The very next day I found I could move the knee much more easily, and by the end of ten days, all pain had left the joints with the exception of the right knee which I understood was badly destroyed.

"Within six months all the arthritic symptoms left, and there was just further joint recovery needed to my right knee which continues to take place.

"There is very little difference now between my right and left knees, and I feel assured that within a short time the right knee will be back to normal.

"I used to have great difficulty in walking one block and wondered if I could make it back again. By contrast, now I sometimes go shopping for three or four hours and don't even realize the time. I am also making good progress in going up and down stairs. Everyone I know has commented on not only how well I walk now but also on how well I look."

Had there been a freer interchange of information between the health-care disciplines, this woman and countless others like her could avoid bone damage and a long uphill fight to recovery.

She is lucky she even had a chance for that uphill fight, for the prognosis of the doctors she visited was always negative.

She did not hear: "Why don't you try a manipulative, or dietary approach?"

Instead she heard: "There is no cure for arthritis. We can ease your pain. We may slow up the progress of your arthritis, but you had better resign yourself to …"

## The case of Mrs J. L.

Mrs J. J. was treated rather bluntly in her quest for arthritis relief:

"I spent two years going from hospital to hospital, doctor to doctor, trying to get relief from arthritis only to be told that there was no help for me, that I would gradually get worse and spend the rest of my life in a wheel chair. Each doctor told me to take aspirin, which was no help at all.

"I had just about given up when I heard of Dr Campbell and the wonderful results he was getting with a diet for his arthritis patients.

"After going on his diet, in two months I was completely free from pain and for the first time in two years was able to go back to work. I am entirely free of any sign of arthritis. There is no need for anyone to suffer, there is help."

All doctors mean well and do their best. But we have a responsibility to our patients that should transcend the barriers of the separate health-care disciplines.

## Gout – uric acid disease

The Arthritis Foundation conceded that there is one form of arthritis that responds to diet. I concede that there is one form of arthritis that responds to drugs. We are both talking about gout.

Uric acid is the culprit in gout. It is not a general pollution of the body as are other forms of arthritis. What causes the body to accumulate larger quantities of uric acid than the kidneys can get rid of is another question. It might have something to do with that very pollution caused by denatured, devitalized, destroyed foods.

Gout was long thought to be the result of high living. Cartoonists poked fun at the gout sufferer depicting him as an affluent, paunchy member of the aristocracy with his swollen foot proped up while he crammed food down his mouth with a bottle of expensive wine standing by to wash it down.

Now it is recognized to be more emotion-orientated, though rich living can trigger it into action. A survey by the armed services of its gout-case records showed that the disease favoured persons of above average intelligence and often struck when morale was low such as when transferring from one post to another.

Later, in 1963, researcher J. P. Dunn reported in the *Journal of the American Medical Association* that executives had significantly higher levels of uric acid than craftsmen and ordinary types of workers.

The pain of gout is legend. It has been described as "molten lead being injected into the joint" and "your toe in a vice tightened as far as it will go and then given one more turn."

## Remedies for gout

Do you know what is one of the most effective drugs for gout?

You guessed it, aspirin.*

One of the many physiological effects of aspirin, besides its reduction of pain, is the lowering of the uric acid level in the blood. Thus it is custom-built for the gout sufferer.

Nevertheless, new drugs are now available to lower uric acid or to break up the painful crystals that form and deposit themselves usually in the joint extremities. Drugs aimed at lowering the uric acid are maintenance or preventive drugs – that is, they need to be taken continually in order to stave off gout attacks.

Drugs aimed at dissolving or dissipating the uric acid crystals are taken only at the time of the attacks to relieve, shorten, and end them. Drugs like probenecid and sulfinpyrazone lower the body's storage of uric acid by encouraging its elimination through the urine. Drugs like allopurinol reduce the body's production of uric acid. Drugs like colchicine and phenylbutazone dissipate the crystals when they form in a gout attack.

Colchicine is one of the oldest gout remedies. It can dissipate an attack within 24 hours. It can cause nausea and stomach distress if taken at a more than tolerable level. The newer drugs are largely anti-inflammatories and are tolerated more easily by some gout sufferers.

## The primary importance of diet

Diet is still of primary importance. Many of today's gout sufferers would probably not know what gout was if their metabolic balance had not been tipped one way or the other by 'civilized' foods.

---

* Remember that large amounts of aspirin can damage the delicate lining of the stomach. Drugs containing ibuprofen can do the same. Talk with your doctors about safe alternatives.

The dietary sources of uric acid are not the basic cause of gout. There is a uric acid reaction to orange juice, to mushrooms, to cauliflower, to organ meats, and to beef. Some seafoods such as shrimp and lobster have a uric acid content. If a person is creating his own uric acid at a greater than normal rate, then partaking of these foods can provide just enough additional uric acid to set off the crystallization process that means an attack of gout.*

The dietary approach to curing gout might be on a more causal level. A number of metabolic defects must underlie the body's overproduction of uric acid. What are the dietary deficiencies that cause these metabolic defects? If these could be identified and compensated for, then a steak or calf's liver or lobster would no longer tilt the scales enough to be noticed.

Of course, neither should we ignore the emotional factors that contribute to the metabolic defects behind high uric acid.

In 1969 the *Journal of the American Medical Association* reported on a research conducted by the University of Edinburgh on 100 business and professional men. It showed that the top-level people showed a higher uric acid content than the middle-level ones. Personality traits that showed a positive correlation with uric acid level included 'drive' and 'achievement.'

The stesses of civilization are often beyond man's normal capabilities to cope with them. They can cause metabolic defects. But man's ability to cope increases with his nutritional level. For instance, a lack of thiamine, known as vitamin $B_1$, can cause personality changes that induce irritability and periods of depression. There are many more irrefutable examples linking nutrition and temperament.

So back we go to nutrition for Mr Gout Sufferer (95 per cent are men) and if the attacks still occur there's always that relief available in the medicine chest. One day – with less 20th-century tension and fewer 'civilized' foods – the attacks may cease.

---

* Nevertheless, it is helpful to avoid foods which have high uric acid content. This includes some of the organ meats recommended in Dr Campbell's diet.

## Some good 'medicine' for all arthritics

Just as certain high uric acid foods can tip the scales and bring an attack of gout, so certain emotions can cause poisons to accumulate which when added to the poisons we feed our body can accelerate the onset of arthritis. There have been many instances in health records of men and women experiencing the initial onslaught of arthritis after a divorce or separation, or after a death in the family, or similar emotional strain or shock.

There are also many cases where such emotional stress aggravates arthritis. Where emotional stress is lessened or eliminated in the life of a person with arthritis there is often a marked improvement in the condition.

I know of no cure based on emotional 'medicine,' but it is nevertheless helpful medicine to take.

As gout sufferers were found to have some similar personality traits, arthritis sufferers have also been 'tagged.' I don't think that any scientifically controlled survey has even been made but small talk among health people points to tendencies among many of their arthritis patients towards stubborn, inflexible attitudes, a lack of generosity, and predominant self-centredness.

One wonders whether arthritis causes these tendencies or is in part caused by them. The picture these traits paint is closely aligned with the physical manifestation.

### Emotional aggravations of arthritis

Emotionally caused problems often manifest themselves just that way. A person with back trouble is often betraying the fact that he bears the problems of the world on his shoulders. "He gives me a pain in the neck" is more likely to give the speaker such a pain than to cause trouble for the one spoken of. The same with other figures of speech.

Emotions and platitudes, are not the basic cause of arthritis. That cause, as you know, is the depleted, denatured, and doctored food we eat.

Still, negative emotions never did anybody any good. Positive emotions never did anybody any harm. In fact, the positive outlook permits nature's healing force to work unhindered.

## A prescription for mental medicine

Here is a prescription for those who want to avoid arthritis or to assist nature to cure arthritis: Take your emotional temperature. If it registers high in anxiety, fear, antagonism, insecurity or other similar stress reactions – simmer down. Learn to ride with life's punches.

Become an amateur philosopher. Understand life's problems as challenges. Know that 99 per cent of all the things we worry about never come to pass. They are wasted effort, wasted strength, wasted good health. Develop a philosophical attitude towards trouble. Think about past troubles and how eventually everything worked itself out for the best.

I'm an osteopath, not a psychiatrist. But you'd be surprised how often a health-care practitioner is called upon to listen to private troubles and how therapeutic such venting can be for the patient.

If you are still sceptical, let me put it to you in a different way:

Everyone knows how emotions can spoil the appetite.
Everyone knows how anger and disharmony can affect the digestive processes.
Everyone knows how bitter arguments can touch off gallstone attacks or how other worry and anxiety can cause stomach ulcers.
So everyone already knows that these negative emotions can interfere with the body's ability to properly use even the best nutrition.

Of what avail then is a perfect diet with a considerably less than perfect demeanour?

- Be pleasant.
- Be positive.

- Be optimistic.
- Feel confidence, equanimity, love.

Easy to prescribe, but not easy medicine to take, you say, especially in the teeth of an arthritic storm.

About 50 years ago, Emile Coué, a French psychologist, had everyone looking in the mirror and repeating over and over; "Every day in every way, I am getting better and better." This was less a case of mind over matter than it appeared. It was a method of reconditioning the attitude from one of pessimism to one of hope and of reconditioning the self-image from one of limitation to one of progress.

The methods outlined in an early chapter to change your eating habits can also be used to change emotional habits. The Coué affirmations are fine and can be worked to fit your needs, but visualization and auto-suggestion are even more effective.

Today is the first day of the rest of your life. What have you got to lose by making it a worry-free happy day?

Give yourself an emotional tonic.

It is bound to improve your physical health.

## A re-statement for self-help

You can restore your own good health by recognizing that drugs and chemicals may not be the medical style to cure a body already over-drugged and over-chemicalized.

The medical style you need is one that purifies the most important fluid in your body – the blood, recognized for centuries as the veritable 'carrier of life.'

You need to remove, replace, and replenish.

- You need to *remove* the poisons that are clogging your elimination system and feeding back into your blood.
- You need to *replace* the chemical-laden foods that are polluting your blood by substituting foods that add no further poisons to your 'carrier of life.'

- You need to *replenish* your bloodstream with the natural nutrients your body must have to permit you to enjoy your rightful heritage of a pain-free, healthy, and happy life.

## For your action

Do not permit tooth extractions or other types of surgery to be performed on you in the name of arthritis cure. Arthritis is not caused by an infection but both the arthritis and the infection may share the same cause.

Keep your resistance to disease high by healthful living habits. Avoid prolonged use of gold compounds, cortisone, and cortisone-related drugs as they can permanently change blood chemistry and interfere with rather than lead to an arthritis cure.

Gout sufferers can use some drugs to deal effectively with attacks. Sufferers from all other types of arthritis must understand the importance of pure blood and take the non-drug steps that lead to the purification of their 'carrier of life.'

# CHAPTER 11

# How to Add Vigorous Arthritis-free Years to Your Life

Arthritis can be cured. This does not mean, however, you have gained any immunity from it. It is only a few wrong dietary steps away. This chapter helps you prevent recurrences of arthritic miseries by acquiring several permanent health habits orientated to a long and pain-free life.

You can be rid of the heat, swelling, and pain of arthritics next week.

You can also join the ranks of pain-riddled arthritics next week. Which of the above choices do you want for yourself? Those of us who do not suffer from arthritis tread a much more narrow path than we realize.

This chapter offers insurance not only to those who are now ridding themselves of arthritis, but also to those who have not had arthritis. I offer this insurance so that you will not find yourself one day off the edge of the narrow path of good health and attacked by arthritis.

I think the health path is narrowing to the advantage of arthritis, and other diseases also, at least in the United States. The chemical balance that provides a proper metabolism is becoming an increasingly delicate one for more and more millions of people in our country.

Recently the wire services carried a news account of the death of 37 soldiers in Honduras after eating food that was sprayed with an insecticide. Forty other soldiers were hospitalized in grave condition at the Tegucigalpa general hospital.

The name of the insecticide does not matter. It happens to have been made in West Germany but had a wide international distribution. There are no laws controlling the use of insecticides in Honduras. There are a number of such laws in the United States because of an increasing awareness of the dangers involved.

It was a quick death for these men.

It is a tortured life for many more.

The President's Council on Environmental Quality reported in May, 1971, that there are at least 14 commonly used materials which are capable of posing serious health and environmental problems. Of course, DDT is on that list as well as the recently publicized mercury compounds. But also in common use are such classically toxic substances as arsenic, lead, and copper.

The Council also warned of cadmium, chromium, barium, beryllium, zinc, vanadium, selenium, silver, and manganese. These are all known poisons. (Chromium, manganese, selenium, and zinc, are also important nutrients known to play significant roles in our metabolism as trace elements. They can, however, prove toxic if we are exposed to them in excessive quantities, such as the repeated use of selenium-containing anti-dandruff shampoos.)

But what is somewhat more alarming is the fact that there are some 10,000 synthetic replicas of organic compounds now in commercial use, many of which have been tested and found to have dangerous effects. Examples cited include NTA, used by detergent manufacturers as a substitute for phosphates until the government showed that it might be a health hazard, and a family of compounds known as PCBs, related to DDT.

The Council wisely pointed out that while toxic effects may be easily observed at high levels of exposure, little is known about the effects on health over a long period of time with low levels of exposure.

I cannot prove that prolonged exposure to any particular chemical substance is the direct cause of arthritis, but I can prove that when persons with arthritis discontinue exposure to groups of these chemical substances, their arthritis can be cured.

This type of 'accusation by association' was fought by tobacco companies for many years. Still, though the culprit could not actually be observed in the act, or cause and effect be scientifically proved, tobacco has been labelled as a potential health hazard. Look at the health warning on any pack of cigarettes.

Whether you have arthritis or not, look at every label that lists the chemical additives in food. Then provide your own additives: the words 'POTENTIAL HEALTH HAZARD.'

## Sidestep the pain of arthritis permanently

A novel by Dr E. Gordon Dickie entitled *1976* features a cancer epidemic and, as described on the jacket, other 'real and unspeakable horrors that await mankind ... unless science can be stopped now!'

But wait, all is not lost. Science has an antidote for its own poisons.

A new technique for controlling pain is being developed. It is based on electrical impulses. Researchers have found that electrical signals can choke off pain signals. It seems that the nerves get overloaded and the entire feeling of pain does not get through. To create these electrical impulses a set of platinum electrodes is implanted in the spinal cord connected by wires under the skin to an electrical coil under the skin of the chest. When the patient feels pain, he moves a gadget to his chest. This starts a current in the coil. It is transmitted to the spine. There it blocks out the pain signals.

Would you rather stick to the aspirin?

Or would you prefer to do without the pain in the first place?

The latter takes some doing. You not only have to be your own nutritionist, you have to be your own ecologist.

Scientific 'progress' is moving at a much faster rate than governmental agencies can possibly cope with. The resulting time lag can add pain to years, and take years off your life. You must be your own protector of your own health, and this book shows you how, with the emphasis on arthritis.

*There is no need for anyone who is recovering from arthritis to ever get an arthritis attack again.*

There is no need for anyone reading this book who has never had arthritis to have to experience its suffering.

All it takes is vigilance and recognition.

It takes vigilance in supporting any new legislation, ordinances, or regulations that slow up the chemicalization process. I'll give you an example of this in a minute.

It takes recognition of where poisons may be lurking in the food you eat and how to 'eat around' them. And I'll give you plenty of guidelines on this score in this chapter.

You owe it to yourself to be alert to anything you need on this subject. It will help you to be your own *practical* ecologist. It will also help you to keep abreast of new scientific developments that might affect your health, developments perhaps along totally unexpected lines in these fast-moving times.

Always keep in mind that small amounts of chemicals, though they show no apparent harmful effects even over a period of months, are actually doing something to your body

Is it something you want?

Chances are it is something you don't want.

You can avoid the pain of arthritis for the rest of your life if you can avoid present and future pollutants in food.

This is something at which you cannot be totally successful. But the body is a beautiful machine. It can correct some of the mistakes of its operator!

Perhaps if the body was less 'permissive' we would be more aware of it and conscientious about our obligations to it.

### Defence against the tricks of the trade

An amateur magician is performing at a party "Take a card," he says holding the fanned deck out to a pretty miss. She selects one.

"Now look at it, but don't let me see it." He closes his eyes.

"I see red. It's a diamond. The three of diamonds."

She nods her head as her jaw drops in genuine astonishment.

What she does not know is that he had cleverly induced her to take that card. He had extended the deck to her in such a way that it would be the easiest card to reach for. Of course, had she known what was happening, it would have been a different story.

*And that's the point of my story.*

If you know that every product that comes into contact with your body internally or externally is a contributor to your good health or bad health, there is no trick to being your own practical ecologist.

Attacks on your natural way of living can come from any direction. New substances are being devised daily. They can become part of your house, your clothing, your cosmetics, your toiletry, your food. There will be new scented air sprays, cleansing agents, insecticides, all of which may aggravate your arthritis.

You owe it to your continued good health to investigate each. I don't mean with guinea pigs. But a letter of query to a company whose product you may decide to 'marry' for your regular use is no 'big deal.' It is worth many times the effort it takes to find out the chemicals involved and the safety tests that have been run.

Newspapers are now publicizing findings almost daily. Ecology, pollution and consumerism are top-priority news stories. Books are being written on the subject that make Rachel Carson's *Silent Spring* all the more a prophetic masterpiece. *Cosmetics Unmasked* * by Stephen Antczak and Gina Mae Antczak and *E for Additives* ** by Maurice Hanssen are the vanguard I am sure of many more to come. They deserve to be read.

If the information you have is not totally reassuring, it is better to refrain now than repent later.

### Two warnings regarding possibilities of arthritis

If you are not exceeding your body's tolerance for the stabilizers, preservatives, additives, and antibiotics that are being pumped into your food when your back is turned …

If you are sidestepping the bulk of the hormones, pesticides, enzymes, and other toxic substances that are put in your daily path…

If you are consuming adequate amounts of fresh, natural foods rich in nutrients…

Then you will be paving the way to continued good health and freedom from arthritis.

* Thorsons, 2002.
** Thorsons, 2001.

If you are not, then you had better watch for two warning signs that are a common 'welcome' mat to arthritis:

Fatigue.
Constipation.

A woman came to see me complaining that she was "always tired." She said she used to be full of energy but now even the smallest task seemed immense. I could see the arthritic handwriting on the wall and gave her an appropriate diet.

Six months later she returned. She had pains in her knees and visible signs of arthritis in her stiffening fingers. I asked her if she had been following the diet I had given her. "No Doctor," she replied, "I was sure my fatigue was due to not enough blood sugar, so I have been taking some sweets in between meals to correct it."

She did the exact opposite of what her doctor wanted her to do for her fatigue symptoms – and the exact opposite of what her body wanted her to do.

Fatigue is nature's warning.

It is as important a warning as pain and often the forerunner of it.

Chronic fatigue is quite often a warning of impending arthritis.

## A hobby that combats fatigue and illness

Seneca, the Roman philosopher, said some twenty centuries ago, "Man does not die. He kills himself." Seneca knew about man's self-indulgence. He saw what a soft life and over-indulgence in improper food and drink was doing to people.

If you become aware of fatigue, respect it.

Recognize it as a warning.

Do something about it.

I recommend that the first thing you do about it is start a new hobby: health foods.

Learn about the most nutritious foods and where to buy them. Experiment with different ways of preparing foods so as to maintain the highest level of nourishment.

Any new hobby will create a new zest in your life. But this hobby will vault your level of well-being beyond belief.

You won't be alone. You will find your neighbours intrigued with your interest in sprouts or in frozen banana ice cream and in what you do with honey or molasses and in your organic garden. They are likely to join you in your new hobby, for health foods and natural living are now the 'in thing.'

## The importance of vitamins

Become a vitamin buff. Acquire a reputation for knowing what each vitamin does for the body, what diseases its lack might incur, where the best food sources are. Your friends will be just as fascinated as yourself to know about such vitamin-orientated health topics.

Can vitamins help arthritis? Are they needed in curing arthritis? If so, which ones? How many? How much of them?

Of course they are needed in preventing arthritis and especially in curing it.

We now know that arthritis can be caused by not eating foods that contain the vital minerals including calcium and phosphorus, as well as the oil soluble vitamins A and D, and the essential unsaturated fatty acids. Therefore to ensure recovery the foregoing substances must be supplied in one form or another.

Yet, we must realize that if our daily diets contain sufficient calcium and phosphorus, our bodies cannot use them without the presence of the oil-soluble vitamins A and D and the Essential Unsaturated Fatty Acids. So, to insure the utilization of these important minerals, the oil-soluble vitamins should be taken as a supplement, at least in the beginning of the arthritis cure.

## The importance of essential unsaturated fatty acids

A word about the role that essential fatty acids play in the body would be in order. Much has been learned about these important nutrients since *A Doctor's Home Cure for Arthritis* was first published in 1979. A considerable body of scientific evidence has proven that these nutrients are part of every cell in the human body. They make up a large portion of the brain – which is 60 per cent fat. They help transport other nutrients and biological compounds around the body: for example, some essential fatty acids help transport cholesterol from one location to another. They also form integral parts of small messenger molecules that trigger and control inflammation. This is important news for arthritis sufferers because inflammation is the cause of most of their distress. By giving the body ample amounts of the essential fats needed to control inflammation, the hot, red painful flares that accompany this debilitating disease can be relieved.

For decades, people have noticed that cod liver oil helps manage the joint pain of arthritis. We now know this is because cod liver oil contains some of the specific essential fatty acids that control inflammation.

Based on their molecular structure, there are two forms of essential fatty acids: omega-3 or omega-6 fatty acids. Nut and seed oils are rich sources of omega-6 fatty acids. Omega-3 fatty acids are found in grasses and green leafy plants, green algae, and animals that live on plankton and other water creatures. Omega-6 fatty acids are primarily found in nuts and seeds. Because these two categories of fats differ in their fundamental forms, they do not conduct the same biological activities. Some of each is needed for a healthy body.

Sources of omega-6 fats are common in our diet. Foods containing high concentrations of omega-3 fatty acids are eaten far less frequently, and food supplements are needed to make up any dietary deficiencies. Oil from fatty fish is the best source of omega-3 fatty acids. Not only do fish live off algae rich in these nutrients, and store excess amounts in their fatty tissues, they also manufacture and store specific forms of these fats that are useful in controlling the symptoms of painful arthritis. These are known as EPA (eicosapentaenoic acid) and DHA (docosahexaenoic acid). In addition to forming parts of the brain and nervous system, these fats form part of the molecular messengers (prostaglandins) that control inflammation. Cod liver oil is not as rich in EPA and DHA as fish oil supplements.

Essential fatty acids are delicate molecules, and therefore highly susceptible to oxidation. Adequate supplies of vitamins C and E (both powerful antioxidants) help protect these nutrients so they can carry out their work.

## Organically grown foods and herbs

Get to know about sources for fresh, perhaps even organically grown foods. When are the apples ripe, the cauliflower, the asparagus? When can we go berry picking?

Get to know what herbs you can grow or which are native to your area. Go on nature walks with someone who is knowledgeable about local wild plants or herbs. Learn to recognize them and to use them. Try growing them from cuttings or transplanting them.

There is a trend to food with more calories per nutrient. Reverse this for yourself. Seek more nutrients per calorie.

No longer are you a sheep being led. You are instead your own shepherd. Your future state of health depends on it. This book shows you what to do and how to do it.

## Another kind of vigilance that pays off

Fatigue can also be an internal sluggishness.

Internal fatigue can be a slowing up of the processes of elimination. This kind of fatigue is self-perpetuating. It feeds on itself. The less efficient the process of elimination, the more toxic the body, the more the fatigue.

In chapter 5 we discussed the bowels, the skin, and the lungs as organs of elimination which must be functioning properly if a cure of arthritis is to be promptly effected.

It is just as important to maintain the efficiency of these organs of elimination in order to stay free of arthritis. Keep charcoal tablets in your kitchen or medicine cabinet as a reminder. Use them from time to time to test how promptly your elimination is occurring. Or use the corn test or beet test.

If undigested charcoal, corn kernels, or beets are not completely eliminated the following morning or within 12 to 14 hours, step up your ingestion of raw fruits and raw vegetables, then test again.

Get those bowels current even if you live to wrestle with the enema tubes. A little unpleasantness of this sort may be the price we occasionally have to pay for refined or overcooked foods.

### Stimulate yourself

You can flush the pores of your skin too. A sauna or steam bath will stimulate the sweat glands and rid the body of poisons in the process. Some Scandanavian countries, like Finland, make the sauna a way of life. Public sauna-bath houses are frequented by labourers and business executives alike. There are separate times or separate facilities for women.

There is a steam room, a washing room, and a room to dress in. The action is in the steam room. It is made of wood. Hot stones provide enough heat to keep the room at about 175° Fahrenheit. Water thrown on the stones controls the humidity while a vent provides fresh air and a means of controlling the temperature.

The Finns like to whisk themselves with birch or linden sticks to stimulate the skin. They arrange their benches so that they can sit higher and higher with the temperature rising with each step up.

Saunas or steam baths are excellent ways to keep your skin open as an effective avenue of elimination. You cannot overlook any such avenue in the increasing struggle to limit body pollution.

Heroes in that struggle are your lungs and your heart. Your lungs pour out noxious materials in gaseous form and replenish the bloodstream with oxygen. Your heart circulates the purifying blood to all parts of the body.

You can help both these organs by avoiding a totally sedentary existence and spending part of every day enjoying some form of refreshing or vigorous outdoor activity.

Remember; I'm not plugging for calisthenics or other types of mechanical exercise. Vigorous, natural motion is what the body needs. You don't have to do 20 kneebends or 10 pushups or 500 yards of jogging to give the body what it needs.

You can walk briskly. You can swim, bicycle, or ride horseback. You can work in the garden or chop wood or build something.

If your heart is beating just a little faster and if you are breathing just a little harder, you are on target. The blood is being pushed around more vigorously while at the same time being liberally supplied with the life-giving oxygen your cells require. Never engage in vigorous activity, however, without having your heart checked by a doctor.

Why exercise monotonously with a sense of futility when there are so many ways to enjoy a few minutes of creative outdoor living?

## How to order at a restaurant

People who dine out frequently have less control over the nutrients they eat than do those who shop, cook, and 'eat in.'

Still, there is a way to avoid 'empty' calories and enjoy a gourmet meal that is as healthfully nourishing to the body as it is to the taste senses.

I have a typical gourmet menu in front of me. Let me see what I'll order.

*First, the appetizers. Escargots Bourgignonne* sound fine. They are imported French snails. Excellent protein and nutrients from the sea. But how were they sent – in a can, with preservatives? I ask the waiter. If they are frozen fresh, that is preferable. The *Crab* or *Shrimp Maison* is served with a cocktail sauce (I visualize a ketchup bottle label with a list of chemicals) but I ask for lemon slices instead of the sauce. *Pâté de foie de la Maison* is, of course, chopped goose liver – splendid, if fresh. Prosciutto ham with melon – sounds great, tropical fruit supreme – perfect, if the waiter replies in the affirmative to your question "Fresh?"

*Soups are a gamble.* I hesitate to ask a waiter to trace the lineage of *Boula, Boula Gratinée* or *Creme Vichyssoise*, so I pass it up. A clear consommé is the least risk with little to gain either, as it is unlikely that it is made from bone marrow

*Skip the soup and order a salad.* Avoid the Caesar Salad unless you want to pick your way between the croutons. Order a tossed, mixed green salad or a special salad of the house. That's what I'll have now. I see it contains fresh Bib lettuce, ripe tomatoes, green peppers, green onions, and what the menu describes as 'exotic herbs.' Oil and vinegar, please.

*Entrées* are fun to order because the choice is large and the risk less.

*Frog Legs Sauté Amandise* contains nutritious protein fortified with an almond butter sauce. *Canard Roti a l'Orange* is Long Island duckling served with wild rice (expensive but nutritious). The sauce is made with an orange liqueur flamed at your table. I overlook the citrus in this case as it is worth its flavour and I know the alcohol will be burned off by the flame.

*Calf's Sweetbread* is organ meat. *Tournedos Rossini*, I discover is tenderloin of beef with, I am delighted to know a topping of *pâte de foie* and mushroom caps. Roast rack of lamb, broiled calf's liver, filet mignon, French-cut double lamb chops, *Chateaubriand* (steak) – all are good dining. As are the lobster and other fish dishes.

*The Breast of Chicken en Cocotte* is stuffed – undoubtedly with a bread product – so if I order it I avoid the stuffing. But since it also has a 'rich cream sauce' – rich in additives – I skip it altogether.

Make mine *Beef Strogonoff*, please, but omit the rice (white) pilaff. For those of you who find much of the above a catalogue of cruelty, carnage, and distasteful exploitation remember that most good restaurants have a selection of tasty vegetarian and vegan dishes. Delicately cooked vegetables, pates, and rissottos, or imaginative salads, garnished with herbs and the cleansing garlic.

*Dessert and beverage* are where your dining out requires the greatest self-control. Melon, fruit, and berries are your best bet. Skip all the pastries and glacé 'delights' and any other sweets.

*And remember – you are not a tea or coffee drinker any more.*

In general the smaller the restaurant and the faster the service, the more difficult it is to order in an arthritis risk-free way. Now you are getting into the world of sandwiches, fried foods, and prepared mixes. Fast-order dining boils down to the hot-plate specials and, of course, the salads and fresh fruits.

Eating out in style is just as much fun as ever. The available choices far outnumber the taboos.

And when you honour the taboos, your body's joints enjoy the meal as much as you do.

### The cases against flour and citrus fruits

The coffee and tea habits are as easy to break as to acquire. Most people find themselves feeling better without these stimulants once they have made the break-away.

Other foods on the no-no list for all time are rarely missed as the healthier tastes of natural foods more than fill the gustatory gap for food satisfaction.

There are, however, two foods that people seem to miss most in their diet: citrus fruits and bread. These foods are described below.

### Oranges and grapefruit

I owe you my reasons for the taboo on these two and in giving you these I may partially relent on one of them.

Oranges and grapefruit are favourite breakfast companions. They are good, nutritious fruits. But I have found that in most cases of acute rheumatoid arthritis, *where the joints are swollen and painful, these fruits add to the patient's discomfort.*

It stands to reason that in less acute cases, although there are no discernible effects, eating citrus fruits must be doing no good for that delicate chemical balance. That is why I don't permit their use to my patients.

But here is where I open the door just slightly as to citrus fruits.

*If the heat and swelling is gone, and has been for a number of weeks,* fresh grapefruit and fresh oranges may be added, one at a time and in moderate quantity on a trial basis. *Frozen varieties of their juice are out. Repeat – No frozen orange or grapefruit juice. Also no canned, bottled, or cartoned variety.*

Even when you obtain the juice of the fresh orange or grapefruit you must be careful. You can do it by hand or with a machine auger but full compression of the entire fruit is not permitted. When you exert that last compression you begin to get not just juice from the interior of the fruit but the oils and sprays on and in the skin.

These substances are not removed by washing due to the porosity of the fruit skin. They are poison to the body.

If you resist that last ounce of pressure in squeezing out the juice, chances are the juice you drink will be a credit, not a debit, to your system.

## Bread and other wheat-flour products

Now as to bread, flour, and other products. And believe me, there'll be no relenting or exceptions here.

Nobody has ever proved, at least to me, that bread is the staff of life. Everybody just eats it obediently.

In biblical times, Joseph stored wheat in Egypt during the seven 'fat' years so that the people would not starve during the seven 'lean' years that followed.

Eating bread may be better than starving. But not much.

Bread is probably man's first processed food. To make it you must have flour. To have flour you must strip the seeds from the wheat stalk by threshing. Then the outer husk known as the bran is removed. Whole wheat flour is made from the rest of the seed but white flour requires the removal of other portions of it. Then it must be mashed, ground, and pressed. At first this was done by hand but then came rounded mill stones and then great tempered-steel rollers. Now comes the kneading and the hour of 180°C, 350°F heat. Result – bread.

Nature makes the wheat berry or seed and then must look on with consternation at what man does to it.

## Dangers of gluten products

There is a growing awareness in the medical profession and among nutritionists that a substance called gluten can be injurious to health. This is a mixture of plant proteins found in wheat, rye, barley, and oats. It is obtained by washing out the starch from wheat flour (so the less-fattening high-protein 'gluten' breads have even more of it than white bread). It is tough. It is sticky. It is used to make adhesives!

*The most serious accusation against gluten* is that it can prevent the absorption of a number of nutrients.

When you eat bread and other flour products, you are in effect making it difficult for the body to utilize calcium, potassium, and iron, also vitamins A, D, and E.*

Need I go further? I can! I can describe the chlorine and sulphur dioxide and other chemicals that go into cake flour and the scores of chemicals that go into bread to make it rise better, hold its freshness better, taste better, and everything except *be* better for your health.

I hope bakers won't take offence. I am not trying to put them out of business. Millions of people are able to adjust to bread and live long and healthy lives. They eat toast for breakfast, sandwiches for lunch, and hot rolls, pie, and cake for dinner. For them bread is a green light for good eating.

Those of us who have ever felt a twinge of arthritis are not among those millions. For arthritis sufferers, *bread is a red light*.

For the in-between millions, bread is now but not forever amber – be cautious in its use, even though your body may be tolerating it fairly well.

## Steps to an arthritis-free life

Following are your guide points in mapping your progress for an arthritis-free life:

You are health conscious.
You are 'elimination conscious.'
You enjoy selected fresh fruits and vegetables.
You like your steak 'rare.'
You even check out some local farms and know where they spray the least and use organic fertilizers the most.
You shun processed foods and stimulating beverages.
You are emotionally phlegmatic and know how to 'ride with the punches.'

* Gluten is the real culprit in bread made with wheat. Many arthritis sufferers find they tolerate foods made with flour from other grains. Using flour made from rice, potatoes, maize, and chickpeas, gluten-free recipes are available for breads, and even desserts. Check your bookstore for ideas.

You enjoy outdoor walks or other invigorating activities.

You are, in short leading a partially pollution-protected life, one that gives you the best chance to keep free of arthritis and many other diseases of our civilized world.

*Still, you may have to do more.*

You may be more sensitive and susceptible to the toxins of our environment and you may have to be more cautious than others.

How does one know?

Aside from the too-late symptoms of pain, one doesn't *know*.

It takes the professional touch.

It also takes preventive know-how.

Standard medical practice, being orientated to the cure of organic disease, finds itself usually too occupied with already sick people to bother too seriously with well people – and how to keep them well.

Annual health check-ups are becoming more accepted by most people, but are still focused on discovering symptoms rather then preventing them.

In some areas of China it has been said people used to pay doctors to keep them healthy, and stopped paying when they became ill and needed treatment. Can you imagine what changes would occur in the United States and Europe if this was our system of health care?

It won't even come for our personal automobile. Aside from standard lubrication and switching of tyres, there is little chance to have preventive mechanical work done.

It pays to take preventive steps for good health for your body. You now know, by having read this far in the book, how important it is for an arthritis-free life. Set your defences against the underground attacks of arthritis while you may still have good health.

## For your action

- Make healthful living your hobby. Keep abreast of latest scientific developments that affect food and water; evaluate them against a standard of natural living versus possible chemical pollution.

- Stick to your nutritional guns in a restaurant.
- Keep a watchful eye on your organs of elimination. Enjoy some outdoor activity every day.
- Don't take good health for granted.

# CHAPTER 12

# The Most Important Chapter of All – The One You Can Write

This last chapter is the most important one of all because it is a new and vital chapter in your life, one that you will indeed write yourself. It is a chapter you will always remember.

It has been a joy to me to have guided the countless cures of arthritis brought about through the simple home methods I have outlined for you in the pages of this book. But it has been frustrating up until now that the word has not been more widely spread in health circles – of every discipline – so that the plague we call arthritis can die a *natural* death, – literally.

Now you have received that word in this book.

If you have been following the arthritis-cure methods as you read, then in the normal time that it takes to read a book – one week give or take a couple of days – your pain, heat, and swelling have subsided, and your bones and joints are on the mend.

If, on the other hand, you have read this book and not yet acted on it, now is the time to launch an attack against the pains and chains of that insidious tormenter ... arthritis.

## "It's like being born again"

I knew a widower in his mid-fifties who looked like he could be 70. He did not have arthritis but he had seemed to live a pained life ever since his wife's death, some ten years before. At a friend's insistence he met just the right young woman. In a few weeks they were married. I saw him some time later. He looked like a man of 35, just radiating vim, vigour, and vitality.

This transformation also occurs among people who have suffered the pains and crippling of arthritis and are all of a sudden relieved of the shackles they had accepted as a prelude to death.

### A particularly convincing case history

This middle-aged man, with one of the worst cases of arthritis I have ever seen, tells the following story of rebirth in more vivid detail:

"I went on this treatment [of Dr Campbell's] as a last resort. All medical men, including orthopaedic physicians, said there was little or nothing that could be done for me. The verdict in most cases was that in a few years I would be in a wheel chair, and in from seven to ten years I would be dead unless I had an operation, had my joints fused, and moved to a warm, dry climate. In most cases they prescribed a pain killer and plenty of rest.

"After Dr Campbell had given me a complete physical examination and ran a series of tests, he said he thought he could help me. It might possibly be a long ordeal, and I would have to go on a very strict diet. This I did, and he was right.

"Week after week, and year after year, following a very strict diet, and getting his manipulative treatments I have finally become free of all pain.

"My case was one of the worst he had ever encountered. My vertebrae had fused completely. Some have become separated through his manipulation. The diet also was an important factor. You have read his book and are aware of it. To this day we follow it, eating plenty of fish, shell fish, liver, fresh fruits, and vegetables, drinking plenty of milk and staying away from candy, cake, pies, ice cream, and soda pop.

"I now play golf, bowl, swim, and engage in many activities that I could not engage in twenty years ago."

Believe me, if this man could begin a new life after this long ordeal, anybody can. What a pity that he had to suffer as he did for so many years. He didn't have this book. But you do.

Multiply his case by millions and it is a pretty grim picture.

> Your place in this picture is what concerns you and me right now.
>
> What are we going to do about it?

"It's like being born again," said a 62-year-old woman patient of mine. "I feel like I am starting a new life."

### How this chapter can become a chapter in your life

Many people read helpful books and never do a thing about it. They put the book down and that's that.

Another book. Very interesting. What else is new?

Others get their money's worth a thousand-fold. They are the ones that capitalize on the information. They use what they read.

There are many reading this book right now who are wondering why I mention this. They are the ones who went on a one-day fast, as they read the first three chapters, and went on the arthritis-cure diet the second day

They capitalized on the information.

Can you put a price on what they have gained?

There is only one difference between these readers who by now are free of arthritic pain, heat, and swelling, and you who are still shackled by it. That difference is: about seven days. You are about to start now. What they enjoy, you too will enjoy in about one week's time.

Finish the book. You have only a few pages to go. But know when you have put the book down, you will be on your way. Prove to yourself that you mean business.

- *Resolve, now, that when you do put the book down you will not eat for 24 hours*.
- Resolve, now, that when you complete giving your organs a one-day vacation, you will eat only fresh raw fruits and fresh raw vegetables and raw to slightly cooked liver for enough days to kiss your pain, heat, and swelling goodbye for good as set out in this book.

- Resolve, now, that you will use the *charcoal test* periodically and when the period for total elimination exceeds 12 to 14 hours you will give yourself enemas to 'keep current.'
- Resolve, now, that even when you begin to feel your young self again you will add only one food at a time, preferably from the *list of 160 best foods in chapter 7*, eliminating that food if any pain results.
- Resolve, now, that you must *never again eat foods made from flour or flour products; coffee, tea, cocoa, soft drinks, beer, wine, or liquor; sugar, candy, jams, and jellies, ice cream, or artificial sweeteners; canned, processed, prepared, or manufactured foods; frozen fruits, citrus fruits (except as noted in chapter 11)*.
- Resolve, now, that you must help your newly replenished blood to reach affected parts through a programme of *daily motion*, aided by neuromuscular stimulation and simple manipulation.

These resolutions are better than a New Year's resolution!

They are resolutions for a new, vitally healthful life.

## How you should begin to feel tomorrow

The home arthritis cure as I give it to you in this book benefits immediately. There is no waiting period of two or three months or even two or three weeks.

In fact, you do not have to wait two or three days to begin to feel the improvement.

Starting tomorrow, if you are fasting today, you will begin to feel:

- Muscle tension eased
- Swelling subsiding
- Heat in joints decreasing
- Pain reducing
- Tight joints freeing up
- Strength noticeably recovered

Every day will bring improvement. In a week or two the misery you once knew will be but a memory you will be glad to forget.

Nature will amaze you as she restores your body in a fraction of the time it took to get that way in the first place.

You will be back on your feet, no longer dependent on others, able to work again. You will watch twisted bones straighten. You will feel decades younger.

## Make a picture record of your progress and cure

Is one of your joints impaired? Is a finger, hip, knee, or elbow painful to move? Have you had it X-rayed lately? Why not do so or get copies of one already taken. Then get on with your arthritic cure with the programmes in this book. Have X-rays taken again when freedom of motion is restored. You will want to show your 'before' and 'after' pictures to your doctor, your family, and any of your present or future friends who have arthritis.

You may even want to take close-up joint photographs now, and then every few days as the swelling goes down.

Full-length pictures will record your total improvement. You will stand straighter, look better.

It will be a graphic story of a hope come true.

### A final warning against extended drug treatment of arthritis

Extended gold-compound treatments and cortisone treatments affect the blood and the metabolism. The only total failures I have had in curing arthritis were where such treatments had taken place over a long period of time.

Intuitively, Miss P. stopped these treatments:

"I had this horrible pain throughout my body. Legs swollen, and ankles, so much so that walking was very painful, and I practically walked with a limp, but walk I must as getting back and forth to work was necessary to sustain my eating and living habits.

"I had been to several doctors, had been given cortisone, had relief in ankles and walking was greatly improved. Lost some of the swelling, then had bad effects from the drug and this bothered me more mentally than physically.

"Changed doctors again, was taken off drugs – that is, cortisone – then placed on two different drugs again. Relief but bad side effects; changed again, more or less the same procedure. Gave up doctors for awhile, then through a dear friend heard of Dr Campbell and thought what could I lose but another doctor's fee.

"I was immediately removed from all drugs; this was the first indication to me that perhaps I had found a doctor that was interested in his patients.

"Then the diet. It was difficult in the beginning, but when you feel it helps, mental guidance takes over and you rigidly stick to it. Also, I learned from cheating experience and it was not worth the miserable feeling of pain. Yes, about two weeks after starting the diet, I was forced to cheat. It definitely is not worth the pain and torture ...

"I am under the care of Dr Campbell and have found that I can do very well without drugs. His treatment is helping me very much, has ended all the swelling throughout my body, and removes my aches and pains ...

"Also, my friends and relatives tell me – I believe due to the diet – that I look the picture of health. I feel 95 per cent better. I am omitting the 5 per cent due to inclement weather. However, I try and succeed most of the time to stay away even from aspirins. I wonder how much medication a human body can take before rebelling."

Drugs have their place. I use them on my patients when they are indicated as a last resort.

*But they are seldom indicated for arthritis.*

## Write your own medical history

Have you ever kept a diary?

It is usually looked upon as an introverted thing to do, something nobody else is supposed to read, and meant only for your own enjoyment.

Yet, hospitals keep diaries. Lawyers, accountants, and doctors keep diaries. In health care, these diaries are known as medical histories.

I have also used letters written by patients describing their experience, not the way the doctor saw it, but the way they felt it.

You can write your own case history.

You can start now by keeping a diary.

First, write down how long you have had arthritis, what areas of your body it has affected, and what treatments you have had with what result.

### The case of Mrs W.

Mrs W. is anxious that her cure be brought to the attention of others. She is using her restored health to work as a volunteer not only at a hospital, but at a mission, a United Cerebral Palsy Center and a deprived area centre. Here is her case history.

"I had arthritis for several years before going to Dr Campbell. It hit every part of my body before I was 40. I was a strong person and very active, and did everything with my hands. I had a husband and four active children. But with arthritis I was miserable and impossible to live with. No one could help me to move because the pain was so intense and my joints were on fire – a light-weight sheet felt like a ton of bricks.

"The various doctors I went to could give me temporary relief or advise high-potency vitamins – by capsule or shots. But each one told me it was a disease I had to learn to live with.

"By the time an acquaintance took me to Dr Campbell's office I didn't care what happened – a wheel chair was ordered at home and I felt that was that. Dr Campbell saw me on a Tuesday morning, examined and questioned me, told me what to eat, and gave me a treatment. Thursday morning I felt it was great to be alive and moving. You have to realize I had absolutely no medication, only the proper diet and the wonderful treatments. Each day made me feel and look better. It's a wonderful feeling to be able to move on your own power. I devote as many hours as I can to helping others. I'm a volunteer at the County Hospital, and several other welfare centres.

"I go every six weeks for a treatment – good health has to be taken away before a person can realize what a priceless gift it really is."

You can make your case history even more detailed and more useful to others. Here's how:

- Use a calendar-type diary.
- Record every meal in detail for each day.
- Record any changes in your health.
- Record your elimination test results and any enemas, hot baths, etc.
- Record what motions you used to stimulate circulation.
- Record any other activities that you believe contribute to your improvement.
- Record the days when photos or X-rays are taken of your condition.
- Record major milestones during your cure – ambulatory, drive car, return to work, etc.

# Further Reading

These books are listed to widen your understanding of arthritis and its treatment by natural methods. Do not be confused by slight differences of approach from the recommendations made in Dr Campbell's book.

*Acupressure Techniques – a Self-Help Guide* Julian Kenyon (Thorsons 1987)

*The Alternative Health Guide* Brian Inglis and Ruth West (Michael Joseph 1984)

*Cosmetics Unmasked* Stephen Antczak and Gina Mae Antczak (Thorsons 2001)

*Curing Arthritis the Drug-free Way* Margaret Hills SRN (Sheldon Press 1985)

*E for Additives* Maurice Hanssen (Thorsons 2001)

*Eat to Beat Arthritis* Marguerite Patten and Jeanette Ewin (Thorsons 2001)

*Exercise Beats Arthritis* Valerie Sayce and Ian Fraser (Thorsons 1988)

*Healing Foods Cookbook* Jane Sen (Thorsons 2000)

*New Self-Help for Arthritis* Leon Chaitow (Thorsons 1986)

*Nutritional Health Bible* Linda Lazarides (Thorsons 1997)

*Positive Thinking* Vera Peiffer (Thorsons 2001)

*Relief from Arthritis* John E. Croft (Thorsons 1986)

*Rheumatism and Arthritis* Leonard Mervyn (Thorsons 1986)

*The Vital Vitamin Fact File* H. Winter Griffith MD (Thorsons 1988)

# Index

A letter n following a page number indicates that the reference is to be found in a footnote.